Oncology

AN ILLUSTRATED COLOUR

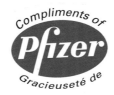

Compliments of
Pfizer
Gracieuseté de

This book is dedicated to our husbands Ronan and John.

For Elsevier

Commissioning Editor: Pauline Graham
Development Editor: Helen Leng
Project Manager: Emma Riley
Designer: Erik Bigland
Illustrations Manager: Merlyn Harvey
Illustrator: Joanna Cameron

Oncology

AN ILLUSTRATED COLOUR TEXT

Orla McArdle MRCPI FFRRCSI
Specialist Registrar in Radiation Oncology
Dublin, Ireland

Deirdre O'Mahony MB BCh BAO MRCP MSc
Medical Oncologist
HOPE Directorate
St James' Hospital
Dublin, Ireland

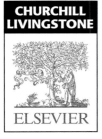

CHURCHILL
LIVINGSTONE

ELSEVIER

EDINBURGH   LONDON   NEW YORK   OXFORD   PHILADELPHIA   ST LOUIS   SYDNEY   TORONTO   2008

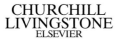

CHURCHILL
LIVINGSTONE
ELSEVIER

An imprint of Elsevier Limited

First published 2008

ISBN-13: 9780443103742

British Library Cataloguing in Publication Data
A catalogue record for this book is available from the British Library

Library of Congress Cataloging in Publication Data
A catalog record for this book is available from the Library of Congress

ELSEVIER your source for books,
journals and multimedia
in the health sciences

www.elsevierhealth.com

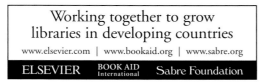

Working together to grow
libraries in developing countries

www.elsevier.com | www.bookaid.org | www.sabre.org

ELSEVIER BOOK AID International Sabre Foundation

The
publisher's
policy is to use
**paper manufactured
from sustainable forests**

Printed in China

Contents

Malignancy in childhood 74

Other sites 80

Oncological emergencies 90

Palliative care 98

Other topics 104

Additional reading and sources of information 118

Glossary 119

Subject index 121

Preface

The modern treatment of cancer draws on a wide spectrum of specialist knowledge, often intimidating for the uninitiated. The aim of this book is to give a broad introduction to the treatment of most cancers employing an easily accessible format and a concise, agreeable writing style. The text is designed to be suitable for medical students, junior hospital doctors, general practitioners, nurses with an interest in oncology and allied health professionals involved in cancer treatment. The large number of illustrations portray typical clinical, pathological and radiological findings encountered in an oncology unit.

Orla McArdle, Dublin
Deirdre O'Mahony, Dublin

Acknowledgements

We would like to acknowledge our patients, without whose generous consent a text such as this would not be possible. Our professional colleagues have provided valuable support and advice throughout this process.

Our thanks to Dr David Delaney and Dr Jennifer Gilmore for their help with illustrations. We are grateful to all at Elsevier for their help and encouragement during the preparation of this manuscript.

Commonly used abbreviations

AFP	alpha-fetoprotein
ALL	acute lymphoblastic leukaemia
ALND	axillary lymph node dissection
AML	acute myeloid leukaemia
ANL	absolute neutrophil count
Ant	anterior
BCC	basal cell carcinoma
BMT	bone marrow transplant
Ca	carcinoma
CBC	complete blood count
CBU	carcinoma of the body of the uterus
CCU	carcinoma of the cervical uterus
CEA	carcinoembryonic antigen
CIN	cervical intraepithelial neoplasia
CLL	chronic lymphocytic leukaemia
CML	chronic myeloid leukaemia
CNS	central nervous system
CR	complete response
CSF	cerebrospinal fluid
CT	chemotherapy
CT	computed tomography
CXR	chest X-ray
DCIS	ductal carcinoma in situ
DFS	disease-free survival
DLBCL	diffuse large B-cell lymphoma
DXT	radiotherapy
EOC	epithelial ovarian cancer
ER/PR	oestrogen receptor/progesterone receptor
ESR	erythrocyte sedimentation rate
FAP	familial adenomatous polyposis
FBC	full blood count
FNAB	fine needle aspiration biopsy
G-CSF	granulocyte colony-stimulating factor
GI	gastrointestinal
HCC	hepatocellular carcinoma
HCG	human chorionic gonadotrophin
HL	Hodgkin's lymphoma
HNPCC	hereditary non-polyposis colorectal cancer
HPV	human papilloma virus
IBC	inflammatory breast cancer
IFN	interferon
IL	interleukin
KPS	Karnofsky performance score
LABC	locally advanced breast cancer
LDH	lactate dehydrogenase
LFTs	liver function tests

LHRH	luteinising hormone releasing hormone
LVI	lymphovascular invasion
mAb	monoclonal antibody
MALT	mucosa-associated lymphoid tissue
MBC	metastatic breast cancer
MEN	multiple endocrine neoplasia
Mets	metastasis
MIBG	metaiodobenzylguanidine
MRI	magnetic resonance imaging
MRLND	modified radical lymph node dissection
NAD	nothing abnormal detected
NHL	non-Hodgkin's lymphoma
NSCLC	non-small cell lung cancer
PCI	prophylactic cranial irradiation
PCR	polymerase chain reaction
PET	positive emission tomography
PFA	plain film (X-ray) of the abdomen
PFTs	pulmonary function tests
Post	posterior
PR	partial response
PSA	prostate specific antigen
PUD	peptic ulcer disease
RFS	recurrence-free survival
RLND	radical lymph node dissection
RMS	rhabdomyosarcoma
ROS	review of systems
RT	radiotherapy
RTI	respiratory tract infection
Rx	therapy
S/C	supraclavicular
SCC	(1) squamous cell carcinoma; (2) spinal cord compression
SCLC	small cell lung cancer
SCT	stem cell transplant
SIADH	syndrome of inappropriate antidiuretic hormone secretion
SLN	sentinel lymph node
SVCO	superior vena cava obstruction
TFTs	thyroid function tests
TNF	tumour necrosis factor
U&E	urea and electrolytes
US	ultrasound
UTI	urinary tract infection
WBRT	whole brain radiotherapy
WHO	World Health Organization
WLE	wide local excision

History and clinical examination

Competent history taking and clinical examination are vital to all aspects of medical practice. A timely diagnosis of malignant disease in particular may save a life or prevent significant morbidity. In the clinic, the findings on history and examination provide an estimation of the clinical stage of disease and provide a framework for further investigation.

History

History taking in oncology follows the standard pattern – key elements in the oncology setting are discussed below. Knowledge of the pattern of spread of malignant disease provides a framework for a logical and comprehensive approach to eliciting the appropriate information.

Patterns of spread

The variety of origin and biological behaviour of cancers in the human body produces a wide spectrum of potential presenting symptoms. A basic knowledge of how cancer spreads is useful. The primary tumour grows by direct extension into the surrounding tissues. It eventually invades the lymphatic channels and spreads along the lymph node chains. It may also invade the bloodstream, allowing tumour cells to circulate in the blood and seed distant metastases in organs such as the liver, lungs, brain and bones. Some tumours produce substances which affect hormonal or immune function. This may give rise to symptoms not directly related to the tumour itself – a paraneoplastic syndrome. A patient may therefore present at the time of diagnosis or during the course of their illness with symptoms or signs related to:

- the primary tumour mass
- involved lymph nodes
- distant metastases
- paraneoplastic syndromes.

The presenting complaint

The presenting symptoms of specific cancers are dealt with in the relevant chapters. An example of the spectrum of potential clinical signs and symptoms is given in Table 1, in this case for breast cancer. The duration, severity and progression of symptoms over time may give an indication as to the biological behaviour of the disease.

Open-ended questions should be used to guide the patient through the history taking process. The history of the presenting complaint should be elicited in the patient's own words. Direct questions will then help to complete the picture, e.g. direct enquiries regarding symptoms suggestive of distant metastases.

Performance status

The general condition or performance status of the patient helps determine whether surgical intervention, chemotherapy or radiotherapy will be well tolerated and is a prognostic indicator in certain cancers (Table 2).

Previous medical and surgical history

A previous diagnosis of cancer may carry a risk of recurrent disease or of second primary lesions. Previous cancer treatment should be documented in detail as it may determine future management. Certain conditions are associated with an increased risk of cancer (e.g. inflammatory bowel disease) and should be especially noted if relevant.

Family history

Approximately 5–10% of cancers occur due to an inherited genetic predisposition. Specific clinical features in the family history should arouse suspicion of an inherited condition. Eliciting and documenting a family history is discussed in the chapter on cancer genetics.

Social history

Tobacco and alcohol are implicated in the aetiology of many common cancers. Smoking should be documented in pack years (one pack year is equivalent to 20 cigarettes a day for one year). Alcohol intake is documented in units per week, with

Table 1 **Symptoms and signs of breast cancer**	
Primary tumour	Painless breast lump
	Nipple retraction, bloody nipple discharge
	Skin changes – peau d'orange (dimpling of the skin), erythema, ulceration, tethering
Lymph nodes	
Axilla/Supraclavicular fossa	Swelling in axilla/supraclavicular fossa
	Pain, brachial plexopathy, lymphoedema of the arm
Mediastinum	Superior vena cava obstruction
Distant metastases	
Non-specific symptoms	Fatigue, malaise, weight loss, cachexia
Bone	Pain at site of lesion with/without impaired mobility
	Spinal cord/nerve root compression due to vertebral bone lesions
	Pathological fracture
Liver	Right upper quadrant pain/tenderness
	Nausea and vomiting
	Signs/symptoms of liver failure
Brain	Symptoms and signs of raised intracranial pressure
	Neurological deficit specific to the site of the lesion
Lung	Dyspnoea, chest pain, haemoptysis

Table 2 **Karnofsky Performance Status**	
Patient status	**Karnofsky performance score**
Normal	100
Able to carry on normal activities, minor signs or symptoms of disease	90
Normal activity with effort	80
Cares for self, unable to carry out normal activity or do active work	70
Requires occasional assistance but able to care for most of his needs	60
Requires considerable assistance and frequent medical care	50
Disabled. Requires special care and assistance	40
Severely disabled. Hospitalisation indicated, death not imminent	30
Very sick. Hospitalisation necessary. Active supportive treatment necessary	20
Moribund	10
Dead	0

one pint of beer being equal to two units and one short of spirits being one unit.

Current and previous occupation should be recorded. Certain occupations entail potential exposure to carcinogens, a well-known example being asbestos. Patients may be entitled to compensation in these situations.

Social circumstances and available support from family members or friends should be assessed.

Review of systems

This section should incorporate systematic questioning regarding potential symptoms of metastatic disease. The presence and severity of co-morbid medical conditions should also be assessed.

Clinical examination

An attempt should be made to stage disease clinically on examination. Clear and accurate documentation of disease extent is vital. A clear description should be given with an explanatory diagram incorporating actual measurements if possible. This allows objective assessment of tumour response to treatment. Pertinent negative findings are as important as positive findings; for example, 'no palpable nodes in the axilla' is of great import in a patient with a breast tumour.

A full examination of all systems should be performed. A discussion of some elements of the examination relevant to oncology is summarised here.

General inspection

It should be noted if the patient looks obviously unwell or distressed. Advanced cancer typically causes significant weight loss and cachexia – a clinical presentation that is unmistakable. Additional potential indicators of advanced disease include severe pain, pallor, jaundice, shortness of breath, abdominal distension, lymphadenopathy and lymphoedema. Reduced consciousness or confusion may result from acute reversible causes or uncontrolled malignant disease.

The primary tumour

If the primary tumour is readily accessible to inspection and palpation the site, size, shape, consistency and

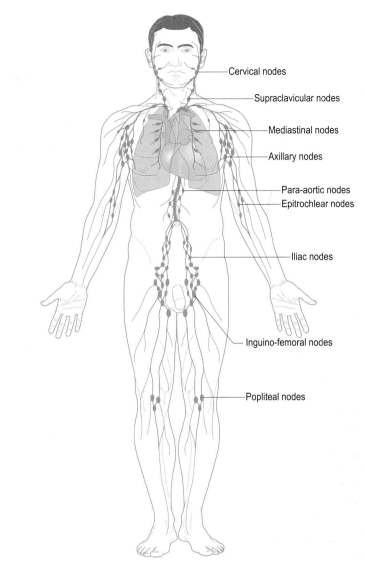

Fig. 1 **The lymphatic system.**

mobility should be accurately recorded. Involvement of adjacent structures and abnormality of the overlying skin are also important. Some tumours are well circumscribed; others are diffusely infiltrative, making it impossible to identify the edge of the tumour accurately.

The regional lymph nodes

Most solid tumours spread along well-defined pathways within the lymphatic system. In general, stepwise progression along the draining lymphatic chains is the rule although so-called skip metastases may occur.

Systematic examination of the relevant lymph node regions allows designation of a clinical nodal stage. A detailed description of lymphatic drainage for individual cancers is given in the relevant chapters. The basic anatomy of the lymphatic system is outlined in Fig. 1.

Distant metastases

The signs of metastases within a particular organ are similar irrespective of the origin of the primary tumour. Some of the symptoms related to common metastatic sites are illustrated in Table 1.

History and clinical examination

- History and clinical examination provide a working diagnosis and an estimate of the clinical stage of disease.
- The extent of disease should always be carefully documented.
- Pertinent negative findings should be recorded.

Investigations

The oncologist has an ever increasing array of sophisticated investigations to integrate into clinical practice. Multidisciplinary team meetings promote the best use of the investigative techniques available.

Oncology patients in particular may require repeated investigation at various stages of their treatment:

- diagnosis
- staging of disease
- assessment of response to treatment
- follow-up after treatment
- assessment of organ function prior to treatment
- management of treatment complications.

Laboratory tests

Non-specific laboratory tests such as full blood count, renal and liver blood tests are performed as routine baseline investigations. Malignant disease or treatment for malignant disease may produce a wide range of abnormalities as illustrated for lung cancer on page 22. These tests are usually repeated prior to each cycle of chemotherapy and periodically during radiation treatment.

Tumour markers

Some primary cancers are associated with tumour markers. These are usually proteins which are produced by the normal tissues in response to the presence of the cancer or produced by the cancer itself. Ideally a tumour marker would have the following characteristics:

- raised in the presence of early stage disease, allowing early diagnosis and treatment
- highly specific, being raised only in the presence of the malignancy in question, not in any benign conditions
- produced in proportion to the bulk of disease
- cheap and widely available test.

These tests may help establish a differential diagnosis and stage of disease. Tumour markers may be predictive of prognosis when raised above a certain level. They are also useful in monitoring response to treatment and diagnosis of recurrence (Table 1).

Pathology

A sample of tissue is required to establish a definitive diagnosis. The technique used to obtain a sample depends on the site of the lesion.

Biopsy techniques

- Fine needle aspiration biopsy (FNAB) – this procedure is performed with a fine gauge needle and syringe at the bedside or in the outpatient clinic. The needle is introduced into the mass and the aspirated sample spread on a slide and visualised by microscopy. The main advantage is speed and convenience, producing a rapid answer when diagnostic. However, the tissue architecture is lost; the cells seen on the slide cannot be examined in relation to their surrounding tissue. This may make it impossible to establish that there is/is not invasive disease present. This procedure is often performed for breast masses.
- Core needle biopsy – this is done under local anaesthetic with a 'gun' which pushes a needle into the suspicious mass. The needle has a cutting edge and is hollow so that a core of tissue is retained within it as it passes through the tissue. This provides a good quality specimen with tissue architecture preserved. Multiple samples are taken from a mass to reduce the risk of sampling error caused by the needle missing the cancer. An example is sextant biopsy of the prostate.
- Excision biopsy – a surgical procedure in which a suspicious lump is completely removed in theatre. This technique is often used for breast masses or enlarged lymph nodes.
- Frozen section – a sample taken during a surgical procedure is rapidly frozen and reviewed immediately for reporting. The findings may dictate the extent of further surgery, for example if the margins of the procedure are found to be positive for disease.

Image-guided techniques

A lesion identified radiographically may not be palpable (e.g. a breast lesion seen only on mammogram) or accessible to direct biopsy (e.g. a lung tumour seen on CT scan). Sophisticated localisation techniques will be required to biopsy the correct area safely.

- Ultrasound/CT guidance – the biopsy needle is directed into the lesion using ultrasound or CT to guide correct placement. This is frequently used to biopsy peripheral lesions in the lung with the needle introduced through the chest wall by the radiologist.
- Wire localisation – used for breast lesions seen on mammography. A hooked wire is placed in the lesion under mammographic guidance in the radiology department. The patient is then taken to theatre and the surgeon uses the wire to guide the dissection. This method is often used in combination with a stereotactic device.
- Stereotactic procedures – these employ a three-dimensional grid which assigns a reference to each point within the grid. Stereotactic biopsy is commonly used in combination with CT for intracranial lesions or with mammography for breast lesions. For intracranial

Table 1 **Tumour markers**	
Tumour marker	**Cancer**
CA15–3 (cancer antigen)	Breast
CA125	Ovarian
CA19–9	Pancreas, cholangiocarcinoma and colorectal
CEA (carcinoembryonic antigen)	Colorectal, breast, lung and others
PSA (prostate specific antigen)	Prostate
Beta-HCG (human chorionic gonadotrophin)	Testicular
Alpha-fetoprotein	Hepatocellular, testicular
LDH (lactate dehydrogenase)	Testicular, lymphoma
β_2-Microglobulin	Multiple myeloma and lymphoma
Calcitonin	Medullary carcinoma of the thyroid
Thyroglobulin	Thyroid

lesions, a stereotactic frame may be attached to the patient's head and a CT scan performed. This allows assessment of the safest approach and pinpoint accuracy in placement of the biopsy needle.

Radiology

The scope of radiological investigations is ever increasing. Specialised investigations are expensive and require skilled radiologists armed with adequate clinical information to interpret the results correctly. Discussion with the radiologist at an early stage increases the chances of a reliable clinical answer while sparing the patient unnecessary tests.

- Plain X-rays – the humble chest X-ray is easily done and may provide an instant diagnosis of lung cancer or lung metastases. X-rays of the bones may identify bone metastases, fractures due to bone metastases or primary bone lesions.
- Ultrasound – useful in diagnosis of breast lesions and frequently employed to assess the liver for metastatic disease.
- Computed tomography (CT) – allows accurate definition of the extent of primary disease, invasion of adjacent structures and enlargement of draining lymph nodes. It is also useful in detecting distant metastases.
- Magnetic resonance imaging (MRI) – superior to CT scanning in defining anatomy and vascular structures within soft tissue or the extent of primary tumour in the pelvis, in the brain and in certain head and neck sites. It is also the investigation of choice for sarcomas.

Radionuclide imaging

A molecule which will be taken up by the tissue you are interested in imaging is labelled with a radioisotope. This compound is injected into the patient's vein and sufficient time is allowed for it to circulate. A gamma camera is used to detect the radiation emitted by the radioisotope, producing an image reflecting the distribution of the isotope in the body. A syringe within a shield is used to inject the compound (Fig. 1).

- Bone scan – intravenous injection of a radioisotope such as technetium is used to image the skeleton. An area of increased uptake produces

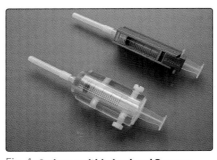

Fig. 1 **Syringes within lead and Perspex shields used for the injection of radioisotopes.** The energy emitted by the isotope dictates the type of shield required.

a 'hotspot' on the scan (see Fig. 1 on p. 99). Bone scans are highly sensitive but less specific – inflammation, infection and a healing fracture may all produce a hotspot similar to a single metastatic lesion. MRI may provide a diagnosis in this setting.

- Positron emission tomography (PET) – uses radiolabelled FDG (2-fluoro-2-deoxy-glucose) to detect areas of high aerobic metabolism, typical of malignant disease. A single scan can provide an image of the entire body, an attractive feature for the patient who might otherwise require several tests to assess the stage of disease. The image produced does not provide anatomical detail (Fig. 2A). The signal intensity from a particular lesion can be measured on serial scans to ascertain the response to treatment. While a CT scan may show a residual mass, the PET can assess disease activity within the mass. It is routinely used in this setting to assess residual mass in nodular sclerosing Hodgkin's lymphoma.
- PET/CT – a combined PET/CT machine can produce both scans in one session. These can be superimposed, combining the spatial anatomy of the CT scan with the functional information from the PET (Fig. 2C). This greatly facilitates the interpretation of both scans.
- Iodine scans are useful in well-differentiated thyroid cancers which take up iodine.
- MIBG scans localise noradrenaline production and are useful in the diagnosis and follow-up of phaeochromocytoma.
- Octreotide scans localise tumours with somatostatin receptors such as carcinoid.
- Sestamibi scans are capable of identifying active disease in parathyroid tumours.

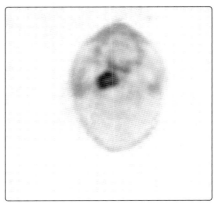

A

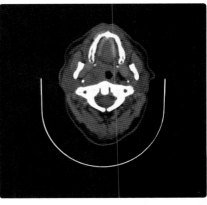

B

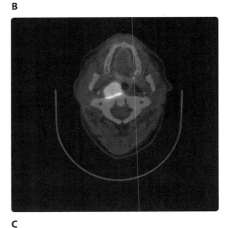

C

Fig. 2 **PET/CT image at the level of the lower jaw.** A, PET image. B, CT image. C, Fused PET/CT image combining functional and anatomical information.

Investigations

- Oncology patients may require multiple and repeated investigations.
- The number and complexity of investigations, particularly radiological tests, is constantly increasing.
- Unnecessary tests should be avoided.
- Multidisciplinary discussion facilitates the appropriate use of specialised tests.

Staging and survival statistics

A staging system combines established prognostic factors to form patient groups with distinct survival outcomes. Accurate staging assists in choosing optimal treatment for individual patients and facilitates informed discussion of the likely treatment outcome. International standardisation of staging systems allows comparison of results between institutions and facilitates the conduct of multinational trials involving numerous institutions.

Prognostic factors

Tumour characteristics which may be associated with outcome are constantly under investigation with a view to refining the staging system to allow more accurate prediction of survival for each individual patient. For many tumour types, the extent of the primary tumour, the involvement of lymph nodes and the presence of distant metastases are strong predictors of survival. These principles underlie the TNM staging system described below.

TNM staging

The International Union Against Cancer (UICC) has published the TNM staging system for many years. Collaboration between the UICC and other national and international organisations such as the American Joint Committee on Cancer (AJCC) and the International Federation of Gynaecology and Obstetrics (FIGO) has promoted broad agreement in published staging systems.

Using the TNM system a stage is assigned on the basis of the following characteristics:

- T – tumour (direct extension of the primary tumour). Tumours within hollow organs are usually staged according to the depth of invasion through the wall of the organ, e.g. colorectal tumours. Others are staged according to the size of the primary tumour, e.g. breast cancer and some head and neck cancers.
- N – nodal metastases (lymphatic spread to regional lymph nodes). The number of nodal metastases, the position and size of involved nodes, extracapsular extension and whether or not nodes are matted together are prognostic for various primary tumour sites.

- M – metastases to distant sites (via the bloodstream). Distant metastases are usually defined simply as present or absent. The actual sites of distant metastases may also be recorded.

All patients are assigned a TNM classification. Patients are then further assigned to stage groupings conventionally numbered with roman numerals as I to IV. For example, a woman with a primary breast tumour >2 cm but <5 cm in size, with negative lymph nodes and no distant metastases will be classified as T2N0M0. Her stage grouping will be stage II. Both the TNM classification and the stage grouping may be referred to as the stage of disease. The staging system for individual cancers is described in the relevant chapters.

Clinical stage

The TNM annotation may include a prefix 'c' as in cT2N0M0 indicating that the stage is arrived at by clinical examination. This designation also includes staging information derived from radiological investigations.

Pathological stage

Pathological stage is denoted by a prefix 'p' as in pT2N0M0. Pathological stage is determined by examination of a surgical specimen after resection of the primary tumour and its draining lymph nodes.

Determining the stage of disease

Many of the tests used as diagnostic tools also function as staging investigations. However, additional staging investigations purely aimed at identifying the extent of disease are usually required after a diagnosis has been established, e.g. a radionuclide bone scan to locate potential bone metastases in breast or prostate cancer.

The number of staging investigations required depends on the risk of distant metastases. For example, a woman with T1N0 breast cancer has a very low risk of distant metastases and imaging of the lungs, liver and bones is not necessary. On the other hand, a woman with T3N2 disease has a significant risk of metastases and imaging of the lungs, liver and bones is necessary to establish the true stage and institute the correct treatment.

The estimation of clinical stage is influenced by the imaging modalities employed. Ultrasound and computed tomography scanning may produce different reports of disease extent. For the purposes of clinical trials the methods used for staging potential candidates should be specified in the trial protocol.

The pathological stage is influenced by techniques used during preparation of specimens. The number of sections taken through a lymph node specimen will affect the total quantity of lymph nodes identified and the likelihood of identifying small metastatic tumour deposits. In the setting of a randomised trial, centralised review of pathology specimens is optimal. Advances in immunohistochemistry, cytogenetics and molecular genetics will allow more accurate prediction of individual prognosis in the future.

Neoadjuvant treatment

Neoadjuvant treatment is increasingly used for common tumours such as breast and colorectal cancer. This allows downstaging of the primary tumour, facilitating subsequent surgery. A clinical stage is assigned prior to treatment. Postoperatively, the pathological stage may differ substantially from the initial clinical stage depending on the response to neoadjuvant treatment (Table 1). It is not yet clear how the pathological stage after neoadjuvant treatment influences prognosis.

Stage migration

The introduction of more sophisticated staging investigations means that tumour deposits can be identified at an earlier stage. Patients who would previously have been stage II using a less sensitive test will now be classified as stage III. This has the effect of improving the overall outcome for patients in the stage III group. This phenomenon is called stage migration and has the effect of improving overall outcome without any alteration in treatment.

Stage migration affects our ability to compare historical patient groups with patients undergoing modern staging protocols. It also compromises comparisons of non-surgical

Table 1	**Case study – stage of breast cancer**	
January 2005	Referred by GP with mass in right breast. On examination there is a 7 cm mass with a single palpable axillary lymph node.	cT3N1MX
January 2005	CT scan of the thorax and upper abdomen are clear of metastatic disease. Bone scan is normal. Biopsy confirms malignant disease in the right breast and axillary lymph node.	cT3N1M0
February–May 2005	The woman receives neoadjuvant chemotherapy. She is examined on completion of chemotherapy. The breast tumour has reduced to 4 cm in size. The axillary node is no longer palpable.	cT2N0M0
June 2005	Mastectomy and axillary lymph node dissection are performed. Metastatic disease is found in two axillary lymph nodes. Postoperative chemotherapy and radiotherapy are given.	pT2N1aM0
May 2006	The woman attends for routine review. There is no evidence of disease on examination.	cT0N0M0

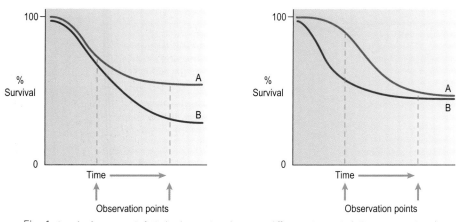

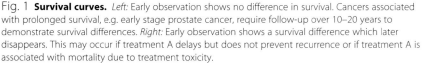

Fig. 1 **Survival curves.** *Left:* Early observation shows no difference in survival. Cancers associated with prolonged survival, e.g. early stage prostate cancer, require follow-up over 10–20 years to demonstrate survival differences. *Right:* Early observation shows a survival difference which later disappears. This may occur if treatment A delays but does not prevent recurrence or if treatment A is associated with mortality due to treatment toxicity.

treatments such as radiotherapy for which patients are staged clinically, with surgical treatments for which there is a pathological stage available.

Survival statistics

Disease-free survival and overall survival are two key endpoints used in clinical trials comparing cancer treatments. The time period in question should be defined in advance. The clock may start at the time of diagnosis or surgery, for example, and stop when a defined event occurs; in this case, disease recurrence or death.

In practice we may not always know when an endpoint occurred, only that it did or did not occur at some point. In this case data are said to be censored. Specific statistical techniques are required which allow for censored data such as the following:

■ The Kaplan–Meier method calculates the cumulative probability of an individual remaining free of the endpoint. Each time an endpoint occurs, the probability is recalculated for the remaining group.
■ Life table method – this is used when the time taken to reach the endpoint is recorded in time intervals.

Comparison of survival statistics

The log-rank test or regression models are used to test for a significant difference in survival probability.

■ Log-rank test – assesses the impact of one variable on the time taken to reach the endpoint, e.g. a particular treatment.
■ Cox proportional hazards model – can assess the impact of multiple variables on the time taken to reach the endpoint, e.g. various clinical characteristics.

The time point at which survival curves are compared may influence whether or not a significant difference is found. Occasionally a difference in overall survival at an early stage will subsequently disappear (Fig. 1). This may occur for a number of reasons; for example, one treatment prevents early recurrences but fails to prevent late recurrence of distant metastases or one of the treatments reduces disease-related mortality but is associated with increased long-term mortality due to treatment toxicity.

Presentation of survival statistics

Survival statistics are commonly discussed in terms of a specific time period, e.g. 5-year survival. The time period is chosen with regard to the natural history of the cancer in question. Cancers associated with a good prognosis require a long time period for a sufficient number of events to occur. Therefore, prostate cancer trials report on 10- or 15-year survival, whereas lung cancer trials often quote 1- to 3-year survival rates.

The median time to the occurrence of an event is also commonly quoted. This is defined as the time taken for 50% of the group to reach the endpoint in question. Survival, recurrence or progressive disease may all be used as endpoints.

Staging and survival statistics

■ Accurate staging facilitates optimal treatment and prediction of treatment outcome.

■ The TNM staging system is the most commonly used staging system:
□ T – tumour
□ N – node
□ M – metastases.

■ Clinical stage is defined on the basis of clinical examination and imaging techniques.

■ Pathological stage is defined on examination of surgical tumour and lymph node specimens.

■ Survival statistics may be quoted over a defined time period, e.g. 5-year survival.

■ Median survival is the time taken for 50% of the group to reach the endpoint of death.

Chemotherapy

The tools of the medical oncologist are predominantly pharmaceutical. They consist of drugs such as chemotherapy, hormonal therapy and biological therapies. This chapter provides a summary of the general principles and different classes of chemotherapy.

General principles

Chemotherapy destroys cells by interfering with the cell cycle, which is crucial for normal growth and development. Cancer occurs as a result of loss of cell cycle control which results in abnormal cell proliferation. The cell cycle is divided into phases by various checkpoints regulated by (1) CDK, cyclin-dependent kinases that phosphorylate cyclins, (2) cyclins – regulatory proteins, and (3) CDKI, cyclin-dependent kinase inhibitors which are negative regulators of the CDK–cyclin complex (Fig. 1). Some chemotherapeutic agents act at a specific point in the cell cycle, whereas others are not specific to any one phase. Regimens often combine agents which act at different cell cycle phases.

To allow for normal tissue recovery chemotherapy is administered in cycles. Each cycle kills a proportion of tumour cells; a tumour of 1 g contains 10^8–10^9 cells, and a cycle causing 99% cell kill results in a 2 log reduction, reducing the tumour to 10^6–10^7 cells. Therefore repeated cycles each with 2 log reduction are needed to kill residual tumour cells. The length of each cycle depends both on the pharmacokinetics of the drugs and on the time required for normal tissue recovery.

Indications

Chemotherapy may be administered in a variety of clinical settings:

- Neoadjuvant – the administration of chemotherapy prior to definitive surgery. The aim is to make a tumour more amenable to surgery, reduce tumour bulk or to reduce micro-metastases.
- Adjuvant – treatment given after complete surgical resection to reduce the risk of recurrence.
- Palliative – therapy is administered with a particular emphasis on improving quality of life.

Methods of administration

Systemic chemotherapy may be administered by mouth or

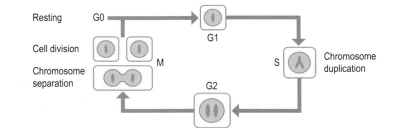

Fig. 1 **Cell cycle and checkpoint control.** Cell division begins when a cell cycle enters the G1 phase; this is required for cell growth and preparation of DNA synthesis. S phase results in genome replication. G2 phase is required for growth and preparation for mitosis. M phase results in segregation of duplicated chromosome.

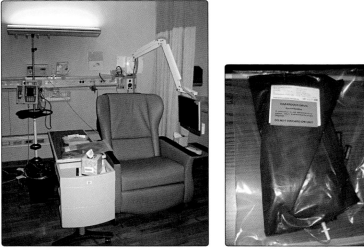

Fig. 2 **Photosensitive nature of chemotherapy/infusional pack.**

intravenously as either a bolus injection or an infusion. Therapy may also be infused into a specific region. This allows higher doses to be administered to affected sites while reducing systemic toxicity. Examples include intraperitoneal infusions for ovarian cancer or intra-arterial hepatic artery infusions. Certain drugs are photosensitive and require protection from light during infusion (Fig. 2).

Chemotherapy regimens

Single agent chemotherapy is rarely curative; it may be more suitable in the palliative setting where a less active therapy with less toxicity is more acceptable. Table 1 outlines the different classes of chemotherapeutic agents.

Combination therapy

- Maximises tumour kill with agents from different drug classes with synergistic activity.
- Minimises toxicity to normal tissue.
- Prevents the development of drug resistance.

Factors to consider when designing combination therapy regimens include:

- use of drugs with non-overlapping toxicity
- use of drugs at their optimal dose and frequency
- use of drugs with non-overlapping mechanisms of drug resistance.

High dose (dose-intense) therapy

Tumours may be refractory to standard dose chemotherapy due to a number of mechanisms including failure to achieve sufficiently high drug concentrations, or resistance. Many drugs demonstrate a dose–response curve; therefore higher doses should kill all residual tumour cells and overcome resistance mechanisms. This approach is associated with significant bone marrow toxicity and requires bone marrow or stem cell support. It has an established role in the treatment of high-grade lymphomas, multiple myeloma, acute and chronic leukaemias.

Side effects

Chemotherapy exerts its antitumour effect by interfering with the synthesis or function of DNA. It is more toxic to proliferating cells. Therefore toxicity

Table 1 Classes of chemotherapeutic agents

Class	Mechanism of action	Example

Alkylating agent	Attach to DNA/cellular proteins preventing cells from replicating	Nitrogen mustards
		  Cyclophosphamide
		  Ifosfamide
		  Melphalan
		  Chlorambucil
		Aziridines/Epoxides
		  Thiotepa
		  Mitomycin C
		Alkyl sulfonates
		  Busulfan
		Nitrosoureas
		  BCNU (carmustine)
		  CCNU (lomustine)

Antitumour antibiotics	Interfere with DNA intercalation	Anthracyclines
		  Doxorubicin
		  Daunorubicin
		  Idarubicin
		  Epirubicin
		Anthracenediones
		  Mitoxantrone

Natural products	Topoisomerase I inhibition
	Topoisomerase II inhibition
	Mitotic inhibition
		Topotecan
		Irinotecan
		Etoposide
		Teniposide
		Inhibit tubule formation
		  Vinblastine
		  Vincristine
		  Vinorelbine
		Enhance tubule formation
		  Paclitaxel
		  Docetaxel
		L-Asparaginase

Antimetabolites	Interfere with essential metabolites for cell division	Folate analogues
		  Methotrexate
		Pyrimidine analogues
		  5-Fluorouracil
		  Cytosine arabinoside (Ara-C)
		Purine analogues
		  6-Mercaptopurine

Others: non-classical alkylators	Inter- and intrastrand cross-links on DNA strand	Cisplatin
		Carboplatin
		Hydrazine/Triazine derivatives
		  Procarbazine
		  Dacarbazine
		  Temozolomide

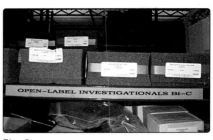

Fig. 3 **Pharmacy stocks both standard and experimental agents for use in clinical trials.**

of cytopenias depends on the drug regimen. Growth factor support (G-CSF) may be needed to facilitate bone marrow recovery and administration of further chemotherapy cycles.

Alopecia

Alopecia occurs due to the effect on the rapidly dividing hair follicle. It is a reversible complication, but often one of the more difficult toxicities for the patient to reconcile.

Growth factors (colony-stimulating factors)

Chemotherapy-induced myelosuppression is associated with significant morbidity and mortality from infection, bleeding and anaemia. A failure to maintain drug administration in a timely fashion can be detrimental to cure. Growth factors are drugs which have the ability to stimulate production of haematopoietic cell lines.

Granulocyte colony-stimulating factor (G-CSF) binds to and activates specific cell surface receptors, stimulating neutrophil progenitor proliferation and differentiation. Erythropoietin (EPO) is produced primarily by cells of the kidney in response to hypoxia, and binds to receptors on the surface of committed erythroid progenitors in the bone marrow resulting in their replication and maturation into functional erythrocytes. Recombinant technology has allowed the production of agents chemically identical to the endogenous formulations.

occurs at sites of rapid cell turnover; such as the gastrointestinal mucosa, Sertoli cells of the testis, hair follicles and the bone marrow. Medical co-morbidities such as liver or kidney dysfunction may reduce drug metabolism and exacerbate toxicities.

Toxicity may be immediate or late.

- Immediate toxicities – nausea, vomiting, alopecia, infection risk.
- Late complications, such as secondary malignancies, infertility, cardiac, pulmonary or renal impairment, can result in significant morbidity in patients cured of their cancer.

Any organ may be affected by chemotherapy administration. The most common acute side effects are discussed.

Nausea and vomiting

GI tract and CNS triggers can stimulate the vomiting centre in the medulla or the chemoreceptor trigger zone to cause vomiting. Correct choice and combination of antiemetic agents with the first cycle of therapy is critical in management.

There are three patterns of chemotherapy-induced nausea/emesis:

- Acute – within 24 hours of chemotherapy; depends on the emetogenic potential of drugs and prior patient experiences with chemotherapy.
- Anticipatory – anticipatory emesis is a conditioned response found in patients with a bad prior experience with chemotherapy.
- Delayed – occurs 48–72 hours after drug administration; it is associated with platinum-like drugs and may last for up to a week.

Myelosuppression

Bone marrow suppression may affect any or all of the progenitor cell lines. The lowest point of decline is known as the nadir. The degree and duration

Chemotherapy

- Chemotherapy describes several groups of drugs capable of killing cancer cells.
- It may be administered in the neoadjuvant, adjuvant or palliative setting.
- Greater response and toxicity are associated with combination therapies.
- The common side effects include alopecia, nausea, vomiting and myelosuppression, although long-term risks of secondary malignancies and infertility exist.
- Growth factors may improve chemotherapy-induced cytopenias and facilitate timely administration of dose-intense therapy.

Radiotherapy

Radiotherapy is useful in both radical and palliative treatment. As a component of radical treatment, radiotherapy improves local control and may improve overall survival. As a palliative treatment, it provides symptom relief and may improve median survival.

Mechanism of action

Ionising radiation produces free radicals within the cell which react with DNA causing various types of damage. The double strand break (Fig. 1) is thought to be the crucial lesion caused by ionising radiation. If a sufficient amount of damage is done, the cell is unable to repair all of the damage adequately. In this state, the cell may die or lose its ability to replicate.

External beam radiotherapy

External beam radiotherapy refers to treatment with a beam of ionising radiation which originates outside the patient. Older kilovoltage machines produce low energy radiation beams which are useful in the treatment of superficial skin lesions. Treatment of deep-seated tumours requires megavoltage (high energy) radiation beams generated by a linear accelerator or cobalt machine.

Linear accelerators

Modern radical radiotherapy is delivered using a linear accelerator – a machine that generates a beam of ionising radiation by firing electrons at a target, typically made of tungsten (Fig. 2). A linear accelerator does not contain a radioactive source. The absence of a radioactive source avoids problems of disposal and exposure to radiation while the machine is switched off. Linear accelerators are costly to buy and maintain, requiring specialised staff to oversee their clinical use.

The main advantages of high energy linear accelerators include:

- Skin sparing – a curative dose can be given to a deep-seated tumour without overdosing the overlying skin. The higher the energy of the beam, the greater the degree of skin sparing.
- Greater beam penetration producing higher radiation doses at greater depth.
- Sophisticated planning techniques can be used incorporating multiple beams from different directions calculated to deliver the required dose to the target area.
- There is a sharp fall-off in dose level at the edge of the beam.
- The beam can be shaped using a device called a multileaf collimator to match the shape of the tumour as closely as possible.

Cobalt-60 machines

Cobalt-60 is produced in nuclear reactors. A cobalt machine contains radioactive cobalt in the head of the machine which constantly emits gamma (γ) radiation. The source is encased in metal and lead to protect

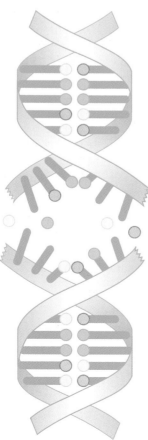

Fig. 1 **Double strand break.**

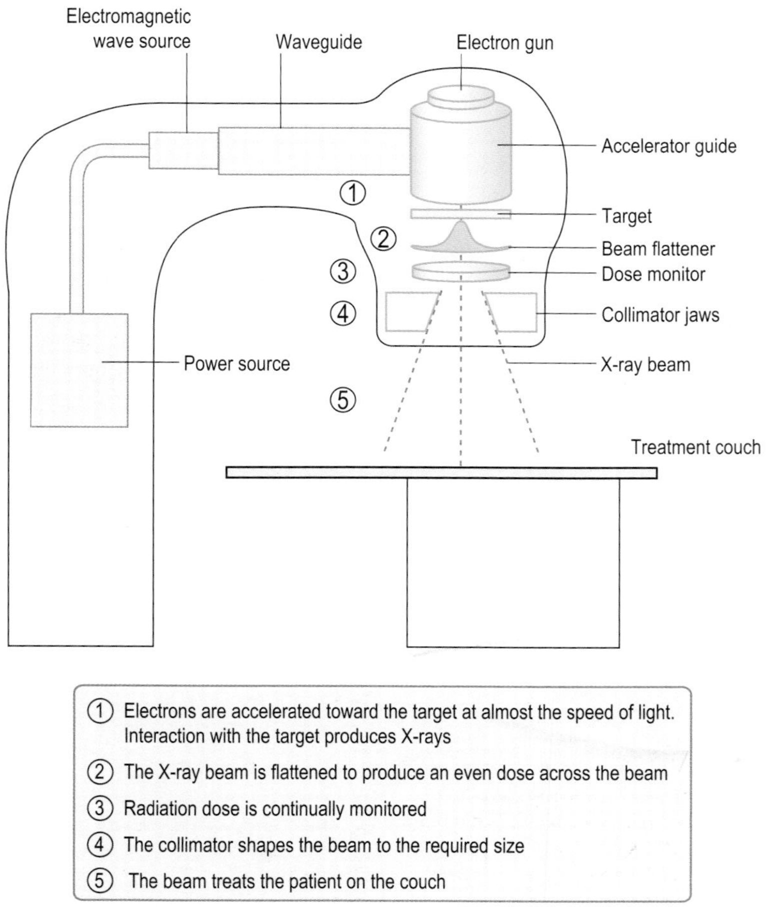

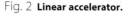

Electromagnetic wave source — Waveguide — Electron gun — Accelerator guide — Target — Beam flattener — Dose monitor — Collimator jaws — X-ray beam — Treatment couch — Power source

① ② ③ ④ ⑤

① Electrons are accelerated toward the target at almost the speed of light. Interaction with the target produces X-rays

② The X-ray beam is flattened to produce an even dose across the beam

③ Radiation dose is continually monitored

④ The collimator shapes the beam to the required size

⑤ The beam treats the patient on the couch

Fig. 2 **Linear accelerator.**

against the radiation emitted. When a patient is to be treated, the source is moved out from behind the shielding, exposing the patient to the radiation. The dose given is determined by the length of exposure.

Cobalt machines are rarely used for radical radiotherapy in the developed world as they are associated with increased side effects when treating to high doses. They are used in the developing world because they are relatively simple machines, which require relatively little technical support.

Brachytherapy

Brachytherapy refers to treatment with a radioactive source placed inside or close to the area to be treated. The radiation emitted by the sources used in brachytherapy is therapeutic over very short distances, which means the tumour can be treated to a high dose while the surrounding normal tissues are spared.

There are three main types of brachytherapy:

1. Intracavitary – the source is placed inside a body cavity, e.g. in the treatment of cervical, oesophageal or lung cancers.
2. Interstitial – the source is placed within the tissues, e.g. in the treatment of breast cancer, superficial skin lesions (Fig. 3).
3. Surface mould – the source is placed within a mould on the surface of the area to be treated, e.g. in the treatment of superficial lesions within the skin.

Placement of the applicator in theatre under anaesthesia may be required. The position of the applicator is verified by imaging (see chapter on cervical cancer). The catheters of the

brachytherapy machine are attached to the applicator in a dedicated room fitted with suitable radiation protection devices.

The machine drives the source to the required position within the catheter to deliver the prescribed dose. This process is referred to as afterloading. Afterloading allows ample time to place the applicator and avoids exposure of staff to radioactive sources. Caesium-137 and iridium-192 are two commonly used brachytherapy sources.

Treatment planning

Radiotherapy planning is a process during which the radiation field and the treatment technique are defined so as to produce the optimum tumour coverage while minimising the dose to normal tissues.

A tumour may be treated with several radiation beams from different directions, calculated to produce the required dose within the tumour while giving an acceptably low dose to the normal structures in their path. During treatment, the machine and the couch move in tandem to the required positions to deliver each of the beams in turn.

- Two-dimensional planning uses radiographic images of the skeletal anatomy to predict the target location.
- Three-dimensional conformal radiotherapy (3D-CRT) based on CT images allows precise definition of the dose to relevant structures with improved tumour coverage and increased normal tissue sparing. Intensity modulated radiotherapy (IMRT), a further modification of this process, produces even greater conformity to tumour shape.

Treatment schedules

The dose of radiation is measured in gray (Gy). Each treatment is referred to as a fraction. Conventional radical

radiotherapy is delivered at 2 Gy per fraction, with one fraction given per day. Breast and colorectal cancer are typically treated to a total dose of 50 Gy, over a period of 5 weeks. Squamous cell cancers of the head and neck require doses of 60–70 Gy given over a period of 6 to 7 weeks.

A higher dose per fraction results in more late side effects, and is usually used only in palliative treatments. Altered fractionation schemes include the following:

- hypofractionation – a reduction in the number of fractions, therefore an increase in the dose per fraction (>2 Gy).
- hyperfractionation – an increase in the number of fractions, therefore a decrease in the dose per fraction (<2 Gy).
- acceleration – the total dose is given over a shorter period of time.

Continuous, hyperfractionated, accelerated radiotherapy (CHART) has been found to confer a survival advantage in non-small cell lung cancer.

Side effects

Radiotherapy produces acute (during or <90 days after treatment) and late (>90 days after treatment) side effects. Any organ included within the radiation field may be affected. Acute side effects are usually reversible, although very severe acute effects may produce consequential late effects. Late effects are often progressive and although theoretically reversible, limited effective treatment options exist. Chemotherapeutic agents such as 5-fluorouracil act as radiation sensitisers and may accentuate side effects. Certain medical conditions such as active connective tissue disease and rare disorders such as ataxia telangiectasia and Fanconi's anaemia are associated with an increased sensitivity to radiotherapy.

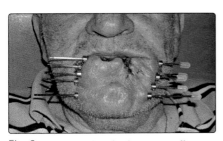

Fig. 3 **Interstitial brachytherapy applicator in place for treatment of recurrent squamous cell carcinoma of the lip.** The radiation source travels through each rod individually. The timing of its movement is calculated to achieve the desired dose.

Radiotherapy

- Radiotherapy is useful in both radical and palliative treatments.
- Ionising radiation produces cell death by causing DNA damage.
- Treatment may be delivered by external beam radiotherapy or by brachytherapy.
- Radiotherapy treatment planning involves a series of steps including simulation and target definition.
- Radiation dose is measured in gray (Gy); conventional fractionation comprises 2 Gy per day.
- Organs within the treatment field may show acute and late side effects.

Targeted therapy

Advances in our understanding of mechanisms of disease have resulted in major changes in the approach to cancer therapy. The identification of specific targets such as receptors, or proteins, has fuelled the development of drugs with a specific mechanism of action, in contrast to conventional chemotherapy which has a non-specific mechanism of action.

Broadly speaking, targeted therapy refers to the use of biological products, cells or proteins. Although there is no agreement on a definition, this group of agents includes hormones, cytokines, monoclonal antibodies, targeted small molecules, antisense RNA structures, and cancer vaccines. These medications have been devised, through the knowledge of their clinical pharmacology and molecular biology, to optimise their effect and minimise toxicity to normal organs.

Hormonal therapy

Certain cancers are known to be hormonally driven; modification of these pathways can have antitumour effects. These effects may be seen by reducing circulating hormone levels or manipulating the hormone receptor.

Much of *malignant breast cancer* is oestrogen driven. The goal of therapy is to prevent breast cancer cells from receiving stimulation from oestrogen. Potential agents include:

- *Selective oestrogen receptor modulators.* Tamoxifen is of benefit in both adjuvant and metastatic breast cancer; it can have either oestrogen agonist or antagonist properties. It may be used in both pre- and postmenopausal women.
- *Aromatase inhibitors.* These drugs markedly suppress plasma oestrogen in postmenopausal women by inhibiting or inactivating aromatase, the enzyme responsible for synthesising oestrogens from androgenic substrates (Fig. 1).
- *Gonadotrophin-releasing hormone (GnRH) agonist.* This may be of benefit to initially stimulate follicle-stimulating hormone (FSH) and luteinising hormone (LH) secretion, then profoundly suppress the pituitary ovarian axis, resulting in a fall in serum oestrogen to menopausal levels.
- *Progestins.* The mechanism of action is unclear. They may inhibit aromatase activity or increase oestrogen turnover, through either the glucocorticoid or androgen receptor.

Prostate cancer is initially a hormonally driven cancer. Androgen deprivation therapy (ADT) is a therapeutic approach for prostate cancer. Anti-androgen therapy can act at several points in the pituitary, adrenal, testicular axis.

GnRH agonists bind to GnRH receptors on pituitary gonadotrophin-producing cells, resulting in an initial release of LH and FSH, and a transient rise in serum testosterone followed by a decrease in serum LH and subsequent castrate levels of testosterone. Anti-androgens bind to androgen receptors (ARs), and compete with exogenous or endogenous androgens, including testosterone.

Cytokines

Cytokines are proteins produced in the body and are responsible for regulating immune and inflammatory responses. Cytokine-directed therapy is being developed as a means of harnessing the immune system to produce an antitumour response.

- *Interleukins (IL).* These are a group of heterogeneous proteins produced by different cells with a variety of actions (Table 1). Clinically high dose IL-2 therapy has been shown to be of benefit in renal cell cancer.
- *Interferons (IFN).* There are three main types, alpha, beta and gamma. The name is derived from their ability to 'interfere with viruses'; however, they also inhibit cell growth and replication. Some benefit has been seen with renal cell cancer, hairy cell leukaemia, chronic myeloid leukaemia (CML) and multiple myeloma.

Monoclonal antibodies (mAb)

The various antibody classes are represented in Fig. 2. Novel biotechnology has allowed the production of unlimited quantities of monoclonal antibodies directed against specific antigenic targets. The process, known as hybridoma technology, is illustrated in Fig. 3.

- *Chimerised/humanised antibodies* are produced using human sequences for the constant regions and using mouse or other animal-derived sequence for the binding region. Less than 10% of it is murine.
- *Fully human antibodies* are produced in genetically engineered mice. These transgenic mice use human DNA to make human antibodies.

Monoclonal antibodies may be administered as a single agent or in combination with chemotherapy. They may be modified to:

- Unlabelled antibodies – exert their action by antibody-dependent cell cytotoxicity, complement-mediated cytotoxicity or even by direct apoptosis. They are specific in their targets, e.g. rituximab – anti-CD20, trastuzumab – HER2neu.
- Radiolabelled antibodies – antitumour activity may be enhanced

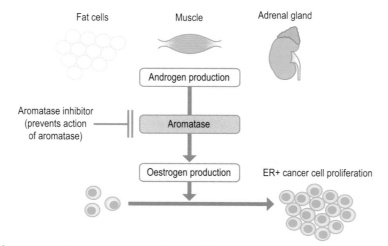

Fig. 1 **Mode of action of aromatase inhibitors.** Inhibition of the enzyme aromatase present in adipose tissue, muscle and the adrenal gland which is responsible for conversion of androgens to oestrogens.

Table 1	**Different interleukin classes**	
	Major source	Major effects
IL-1	Macrophages	Stimulation of T cells and antigen-presenting cells B-cell growth and antibody production Promotes haematopoiesis (blood cell formation)
IL-2	Activated T cells	Proliferation of activated T cells
IL-3	T lymphocytes	Growth of blood cell precursors
IL-4	T cells and mast cells	B-cell proliferation IgE production
IL-5	T cells and mast cells	Eosinophil growth
IL-6	Activated T cells	Synergistic effects with IL-1 or TNFα
IL-7	Thymus and bone marrow stromal cells	Development of T-cell and B-cell precursors
IL-8	Macrophages	Chemo-attracts neutrophils
IL-9	Activated T cells	Promotes growth of T cells and mast cells
IL-10	Activated T cells, B cells and monocytes	Inhibits inflammatory and immune responses
IL-11	Stromal cells	Synergistic effects on haematopoiesis
IL-12	Macrophages, B cells	Promotes T_H1 cells while suppressing T_H2 functions
IL-13	T_H2 cells	Similar to IL-4 effects
IL-15	Epithelial cells and monocytes	Similar to IL-2 effects
IL-16	CD8 T cells	Chemo-attracts CD4 T cells
IL-17	Activated memory T cells	Promotes T-cell proliferation
IL-18	Macrophages	Induces IFNγ production

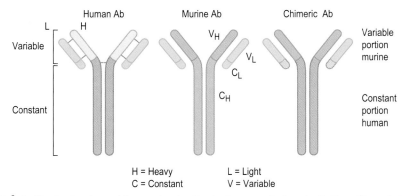

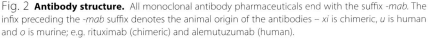

Fig. 2 **Antibody structure.** All monoclonal antibody pharmaceuticals end with the suffix -*mab*. The infix preceding the -*mab* suffix denotes the animal origin of the antibodies – *xi* is chimeric, *u* is human and *o* is murine; e.g. rituximab (chimeric) and alemutuzumab (human).

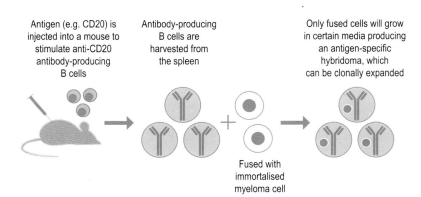

Fig. 3 **Monoclonal antibody production.**

by conjugating the antibody to a radionuclide such as yttrium or iodine, e.g. iodine-131 tositumomab.

- Immunotoxin – antibodies may be conjugated to highly potent toxins such as *Pseudomonas* exotoxin.

Small molecules

'Small molecule' drugs block specific enzyme pathways and growth factor receptors. Protein tyrosine kinase (TK) is one such pathway; imatinib, a TK inhibitor, has been shown to be effective in gastrointestinal stromal tumour (GIST) and CML.

Antisense RNA structures

Antisense techniques are used to deactivate disease-causing or undesirable genes so that they cannot produce harmful or unwanted proteins. Oblimersen sodium turns off the production of Bcl-2, which makes cancer cells more sensitive to chemotherapy. It has been investigated in many cancers including follicular

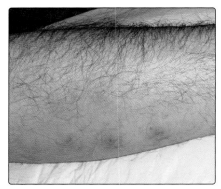

Fig. 4 **Vaccine injection sites.** Vaccine was administered with six subcutaneous injections; a delayed hypersensitivity response was noted.

lymphoma, chronic lymphocytic leukaemia (CLL) and lung cancer.

Cancer vaccines

Potential roles for vaccines include passive or active specific immunotherapy. With passive immunotherapy, the goal is to stimulate the immune system using exogenous cytokines, antibodies, immune cells or growth factors. In active immunotherapy, a specific tumour-associated antigen elicits an endogenous immune or antitumour response. Vaccines may be administered subcutaneously, intradermally or intramuscularly. Injection reactions vary depending not only on the injection type but also on the immune status of the patient (Fig. 4).

The benefit of therapeutic cancer vaccines has yet to be confirmed. However, they have many theoretical advantages; they:

- increase an immunogenic response to the tumour
- target specific tumour antigens
- are non-toxic
- may be combined with conventional therapies and/or other immunotherapies
- may elicit immunological memory to prevent re-emergence of the tumour.

Targeted therapy

- The realm of targeted therapy is constantly evolving.
- The key is identification of available specific targets.
- The effectiveness of monoclonal antibody therapy has been established.
- Several haematological cancers have shown response to interferon-alpha.
- IL-2 therapy has been useful in renal cell cancer.

Surgical oncology

En bloc surgical resection of the primary tumour and its regional lymph nodes is an integral part of curative treatment for most solid tumours. The surgical oncologist may operate to establish the diagnosis, treat the patient or provide palliation. The aim of modern oncological surgery is to effect cure while optimising function and cosmetic outcome.

The best possible results are obtained when patients are treated by specialists performing a sufficient number of procedures per year in a referral centre with the full complement of oncology services. Institutional audit of outcome and complication rate is standard practice.

Surgical practice, akin to medical and radiation oncology, is subject to the rigours of evidence-based medicine. Research is aimed not only at perfecting surgical outcomes but at optimising the combination of surgery with chemotherapy and radiotherapy. The timing, as opposed to the content, of combined modality treatment may have a significant impact on outcome and is the subject of continuous study. Commonly used combinations are illustrated in Fig. 1.

Carefully conducted clinical studies may significantly alter the approach to specific conditions.

- *Breast cancer.* Historically the Halsted mastectomy, an extensive and mutilating operation, was performed. The realisation that breast cancer is a systemic disease and a wish to give women better cosmetic outcomes stimulated the development of breast-conserving surgical techniques. It is now proven that breast-conserving surgery

combined with radiotherapy achieves survival results equivalent to mastectomy and with a superior cosmetic result.
- *Anal canal cancer.* Traditionally abdominoperineal resection with permanent colostomy (Fig. 2) offered the only chance of cure. Complete resolution of tumour after chemoradiotherapy prompted studies which resulted in a new standard of care. Surgery is now reserved for tumours which fail to respond to chemoradiotherapy or subsequently recur.
- *Rectal cancer.* Improving surgical technique by introducing standardised total mesorectal excision has reduced the recurrence rate in rectal cancer. This benefit from improved surgery was maintained in patients who also received radiotherapy, underlining the importance of optimising surgical technique and combining optimal surgery with adjuvant treatments.

Sentinel lymph node biopsy

Many cancers are known to spread step by step to successive lymph nodes. Therefore if the first node in the chain is not involved by cancer, it may be assumed that all the nodes are negative. If the first node is positive, the distal nodes must be examined to establish if they are involved. The first node in the sequence is referred to as the sentinel lymph node.

Sentinel node biopsy avoids the need for full lymph node dissection in patients with a negative sentinel node. In the case of breast cancer patients, lymphoedema of the arm, a complication of axillary lymph node

dissection, can be avoided in patients with a negative sentinel lymph node biopsy. The quality of the procedure is operator dependent – in the hands of a specialist the false negative rate should be <5%.

Method

A blue dye or radioactive tracer or both are injected around the tumour and given time to flow through the lymphatic channels. The dye can be readily seen as it coalesces in the sentinel node as illustrated in Fig. 3. The radioactive substance is tracked with a Geiger counter probe, the node producing the highest reading being the sentinel node. The identified node is removed and the radioactivity reading repeated to confirm that the correct node has been removed. In practice these methods usually identify a small group of two or three nodes. The procedure should be performed before the primary tumour is tampered with to avoid alteration in lymphatic flow as a result of surgical intervention.

Reconstructive surgery

Reconstructive surgical techniques are used to ameliorate the cosmetic and functional deficits which may result from radical resection procedures, particularly in head and neck, breast and skin cancer treatment. Grafting techniques such as those discussed below may be used to replace skin and soft tissue. Bone may be replaced by artificial materials or by bone graft, taken from the fibula for example.

Reconstructive procedures may require extensive, lengthy operations. Failure of the graft may occur in addition to the conventional

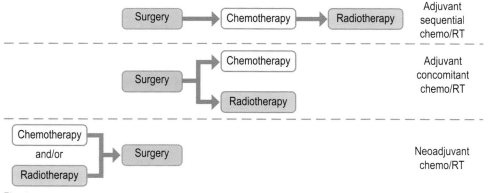

Fig. 1 **The timing of combined modality treatment.**

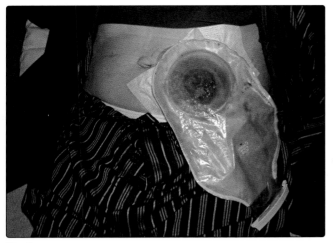

Fig. 2 **Colostomy.**

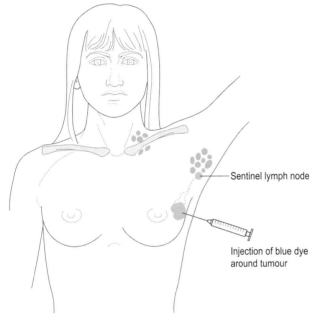

Sentinel lymph node

Injection of blue dye
around tumour

Fig. 3 **Sentinel lymph node biopsy.**

complications of surgery such as infection and bleeding. The patient should have realistic expectations regarding the results of reconstruction prior to surgery.

Skin graft techniques

All of these procedures involve removing skin and/or other tissues from a donor site and transferring it to a recipient site to repair a defect. There are three main types of skin graft procedures:

Split-thickness skin graft. The top layer of the skin (the epidermis and part of the dermis) is removed from the donor site using an instrument called a dermatome. A blood supply will develop over time at the recipient site allowing the graft to 'take'. Meshing refers to the creation of multiple holes or slits in the skin graft. This allows the graft to be stretched to cover a larger area and prevents collection of fluid underneath the graft, improving the chances that the graft will take. The donor site will heal with little difficulty. Donor sites are chosen in areas that are not

usually visible (such as the inner thigh, buttocks and upper arm) with consideration of colour matching in the recipient area.

Full-thickness skin graft. An entire area of skin is removed from the donor site. Cosmetic results may be superior when compared to split-thickness skin grafting. The wound at the donor site usually requires stitches.

Myocutaneous flaps. Skin, muscle and fat with an attached blood supply can be transferred to the recipient site to correct a three-dimensional deficit. Examples include the use of transverse rectus abdominis myocutaneous flaps (TRAM) in breast reconstruction. Free flaps are completely removed from the donor site with an identified artery and vein. Microsurgical techniques employing powerful magnifying equipment allow the blood vessels to be reconnected at the new site. Rotational flaps are left attached to their blood supply and positioned to cover the defect.

Breast reconstruction

Breast reconstruction is a complex field combining the use of implants, expanders and graft procedures to achieve the best results for individual patients. Mastectomy and reconstruction may be carried out during a single operation. Women who undergo radiation therapy may have an inferior cosmetic outcome and are more likely to experience complications following reconstruction.

- *Implants and expanders.* An implant is a small packet filled with saline or silicone gel. An expander is similar to a saline implant with a port attached that allows the surgeon to inject saline periodically. This stretches the overlying skin, producing the required size and shape without the need for further surgery. An expander can be removed and replaced with an implant when expansion is complete. Permanent expanders double as implants and can be left in place when the port is removed. Implants may be used with myocutaneous flaps to produce the desired appearance.
- *TRAM flap.* The transverse rectus abdominis muscle is dissected with abdominal skin and fatty tissue. The flap is then tunnelled under the skin to the required position on the chest wall. The TRAM flap approximates the natural texture of the breast wall but has no sensation. A transverse abdominal scar marks the site of removal of skin and soft tissue.
- *Latissimus dorsi flap.* The latissimus dorsi muscle is dissected and brought around to the anterior chest wall under the skin to form the breast shape.

Surgical oncology

- Surgery is part of curative treatment for most solid tumours.
- The aim of surgery is to remove the tumour with an adequate margin while preserving function and cosmetic outcome.

- Radical resection involves en bloc resection of the tumour and its associated draining lymph nodes.
- Reconstructive procedures may restore function and significantly improve cosmetic outcome.

Breast cancer

Breast cancer is the most commonly diagnosed non-skin cancer malignancy in females, with over 40 000 new cases identified annually. More than 12 000 women in the UK will die each year. A woman has a 12% lifetime risk of developing breast cancer and a 3.5% chance of dying of it. The median age for diagnosis is between 60 and 65 years.

Aetiology

Most women with breast cancer have no known predisposition. Established risk factors are listed in Box 1. Many of these factors relate to oestrogen exposure. Repeated unopposed differentiation of terminal ducts within the breast may allow accrual of genetic hits eventually resulting in malignant change.

Mutations in the *BRCA1* and *BRCA2* genes on chromosomes 17 and 13 respectively confer a 40–85% lifetime risk of developing breast cancer. These mutations are more common in women of Jewish ancestry. Women with a previous breast cancer have a three- to four-fold increased risk of developing cancer in the contralateral breast, equivalent to a risk of 1% per year.

Clinical presentation

Patients will typically present with a palpable breast lump or a radiographically identified mass. In a primary care practice only 10% of patients presenting with a breast lump will be diagnosed with cancer. However, a new breast mass in a woman over 50 years should be considered malignant until proven otherwise. The length of time the lump has been present, changes over time, relationship with the menstrual cycle and abnormalities of the overlying skin should be noted. Associated symptoms may include breast pain and unilateral bloody nipple discharge.

Pathology

Breast cancer screening has resulted in the increased cancer detection. DCIS is described as proliferation of malignant epithelial cells confined to the mammary ducts without evidence of invasion through the basement membrane. It is considered a precursor neoplastic lesion. LCIS tends to be diffusely distributed throughout both breasts. It is considered a risk factor for breast cancer, not a precursor lesion.

The pathological classification and grading of invasive cancers are shown in Box 2 and Table 1. Lobular carcinoma presents with bilateral tumours in 20% of cases and has a tendency to be multicentric. Less common breast neoplasms include phyllodes tumours (cystosarcoma phyllodes), angiosarcoma and lymphoma. Phyllodes tumours are composed of a mixture of hypercellular stroma and benign ductal structures; they may be cytologically bland or frankly sarcomatous.

Immunohistochemistry will identify oestrogen or progesterone receptors and HER2neu expression. The Nottingham Prognostic Index is a scoring system for attributing breast cancers low, moderate or high risk of recurrence. It is based on the tumour size, tumour grade and the number of lymph nodes involved.

Diagnosis and staging

Triple assessment combines clinical examination, radiological findings and fine needle aspiration and is ideally performed in a single visit to a dedicated breast clinic.

Mammography will detect more than 90% of breast cancers in women >50 years. Features suggestive of malignancy include irregular spiculated lesions or linear, branching microcalcifications (Fig. 1). The density of breast tissue in younger patients may obscure non-calcified soft tissue malignancies (Fig. 2). Although CT imaging can identify breast lesions, sensitivity and specificity are limited. Recent data support the use of contrast-enhanced breast magnetic resonance imaging (MRI) for investigation of breast cancer in high-risk young women. Breast ultrasound will differentiate between a solid or cystic lesion.

Aspiration of a benign cyst may reveal non-bloody fluid and often disappearance of the lesion; however, the fluid should always be examined cytologically. Fine needle aspiration (FNA) is a simple method for obtaining material for cytological examination but may be operator dependent. If FNA is non-diagnostic, the patient should proceed to a core biopsy. In the case of a non-palpable mass, diagnosis requires either an ultrasound-guided core biopsy or a stereotactic-guided core biopsy. The latter procedure consists of a specialised mammographic machine and stereotactic table allowing for accurate localisation in three dimensions.

The TNM classification (Fig. 3) system does not account for prognostic

Box 1 Risk factors

- Age >60 years
- Early menarche (<12 years)
- Late menopause (>55 years)
- Late parity (>30 years)
- Oral contraception use
- Hormone replacement therapy
- Personal history of breast cancer
- Family history of breast cancer
- Benign proliferative lesions

Box 2 Pathology of invasive carcinomas

- Ductal 70–80%
- Lobular 5–10%
- Tubular 10–20%
- Medullary 5–10%
- Mucinous/colloid 1–2%
- Other 1–2%
  micropapillary, metaplastic, adenoid cystic, Paget's disease

Table 1 **Grading pathology**	
Grade I (well differentiated)	Cells infiltrate stroma as solid nests and glands with relatively uniform nuclei, no mitosis
Grade II (moderately differentiated)	Cells infiltrate as solid nests with some glandular differentiation, some nuclear pleomorphism and a moderate mitotic rate
Grade III (poorly differentiated)	Solid nests of neoplastic cells without evidence of gland formation and marked nuclear atypia with considerable mitotic activity

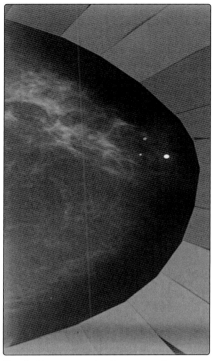

Fig. 1 **Mammography demonstrating spiculated appearance with microcalcification.**

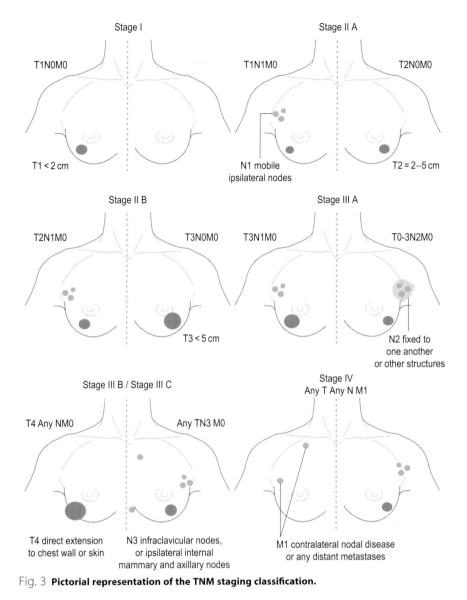

Fig. 3 **Pictorial representation of the TNM staging classification.**

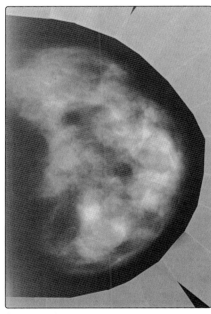

Fig. 2 **Mammography demonstrating the limitations in young women with dense breasts.**

indicators such as hormone receptor or HER2neu receptor status. Complete blood count, liver function test and bone profiles may help exclude metastatic disease. In general, tumour markers have no role in the initial diagnosis or screening of women with early stage breast cancer. Tumour markers may be used to monitor disease in those with known metastatic disease, when no other means of assessing disease is available.

Staging investigations such as radionuclide bone scan and CT imaging should be reserved for high-risk cases.

Management

Management requires a multidisciplinary team approach combining modalities such as surgery, chemotherapy, hormonal therapy and radiotherapy. Treatment approaches vary according to the stage of disease: carcinoma in situ, early stage breast cancer (stage I and II), locally advanced and inflammatory breast cancer (stage III) and metastatic breast cancer (stage IV).

Breast cancer

Breast cancer is the most commonly diagnosed non-skin cancer in women.

■ More than 12 000 women in the UK will die each year.

■ Age, oestrogen exposure and family history are significant risk factors.

■ Mammographic screening has increased cancer detection.

■ Ductal carcinoma accounts for 70–80% of breast cancers.

■ Lobular carcinoma has a tendency to multifocal and bilateral disease.

Carcinoma in situ and early breast cancer

Ductal carcinoma in situ (DCIS)

This is a non-invasive precancerous lesion. It comprises a heterogeneous group of histopathological lesions. Comedo type DCIS appears to be associated with a greater malignant potential. One third of patients will have multicentric disease. Management is primarily surgical, with the choice of mastectomy versus breast-conserving surgery and radiotherapy. Tamoxifen has been shown to reduce both ipsilateral invasive breast cancer and contralateral breast cancers.

Lobular carcinoma in situ (LCIS)

LCIS is not premalignant. The presence of LCIS is a marker that identifies individuals at risk of developing breast cancer. The risk of developing an invasive breast cancer is 8–11 times that of the general population. LCIS is generally multicentric and frequently bilateral. Most women can be managed without additional therapy after diagnostic biopsy; there is no evidence to show that re-excision to obtain clear margins is of any benefit. Tamoxifen has been shown to decrease the risk of subsequent breast cancers.

Early breast cancer

Surgery

Options for surgical management of the primary tumour include breast-conserving surgery plus radiation therapy, mastectomy and reconstruction, and mastectomy alone. Randomised prospective trials have demonstrated equal efficacy. Selection of the local surgical approach depends on the size and location of the lesion, the size of the breast and the patients' preferences with regard to preserving the breast (Fig. 1). Breast-conserving techniques include lumpectomy, quadrantectomy and segmental mastectomy. However, the presence of multifocal disease in the breast or a connective tissue disease which would contraindicate adjuvant radiation therapy are relative contraindications to breast-conserving surgery (Box 1).

Surgical staging of the axilla should be performed. The sentinel lymph node (SLN) is the first draining lymph node from the breast. Methods of SLN sampling have been developed using blue dye or technetium. The SLN is immediately examined to identify any metastasis. It the SLN is negative, no further surgery is required; however, if the SLN is positive, possible treatment options include complete axillary node dissection or adjuvant axillary radiation.

Radiotherapy

For patients undergoing breast-conserving surgery, the addition of radiotherapy is now standard care. Treatment is given to the remaining breast tissue. If the SLN is involved and the patient has not undergone a complete axillary dissection, she should receive regional nodal irradiation. Adjuvant radiotherapy is recommended in post-mastectomy patients with positive surgical margins, a primary tumour greater than 5 cm or involvement of four or more lymph nodes. Radiotherapy is generally given after completion of adjuvant chemotherapy; it may not be given concurrently

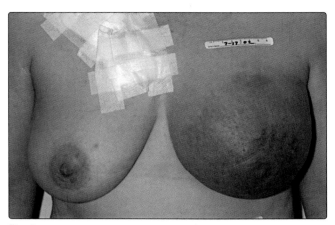

Fig. 1 **Swollen, tender left breast with evidence of recent excision biopsy superior to nipple.**

Box 1 Indications for mastectomy: relative contraindications to breast-conserving surgery

- Patient preference
- Medical contraindication to radiotherapy
- Pregnancy
- Anticipated poor cosmetic result
- Diffuse or multifocal disease
- Extensively positive margins

Table 1 **Response to hormonal therapy according to ER and PR status**

ER	PR	Response rate
+	+	78%
+	–	34%
–	+	45%
–	–	10%

with anthracycline-based regimens due to the radio-sensitising effect of the drug.

Hormonal therapy

The goal of hormonal therapy is to prevent tumour cells from receiving stimulation from oestrogen. This results in apoptosis of the malignant cell line. All patients whose breast cancer is ER or PR positive, irrespective of patient age, menopausal status, lymph node involvement or tumour size, should be offered hormonal therapy (Table 1). The primary source of oestrogen in the premenopausal woman is the ovary, while in postmenopausal women it is the peripheral conversion of adrenal androgens to oestrogen by the enzyme aromatase. Hormonal blockade may be attained by blocking the hormone receptor or by inhibiting aromatase.

Chemotherapy

Both pre- and postmenopausal women benefit from adjuvant chemotherapy. Anthracycline-based chemotherapy is superior to non-anthracycline-based chemotherapy. Overall adjuvant chemotherapy reduces the risk of recurrence by 25%. Adjuvant chemotherapy is routinely offered to women with a primary tumour that is 1 cm or larger. Within the subset of patients with a tumour less than 1 cm or node negative the benefit is uncertain.

The optimal sequence of therapy is uncertain; the standard approach is to start adjuvant chemotherapy 3–6 weeks after surgery, with the administration of radiotherapy after this period. It has been shown that patients who received chemotherapy first have an improvement in overall survival, local and distant recurrence rates.

Up to 20% of breast cancers have amplification or over-expression of the gene encoding the cell surface molecule HER2neu, a member of the epidermal growth factor receptor family. This is predictive of benefit with anti-HER2neu-directed therapy.

Recent data suggest benefit of Herceptin therapy, a monoclonal antibody against HER2neu, in the management of early breast cancer.

Male breast cancer

One per cent of all breast cancers are identified in men. The median age at diagnosis is 65 years. Similar to female breast cancer it is a hormonally driven cancer; therefore it is found in men with relative oestrogen excesses due to endogenous production such as in Klinefelter's syndrome, chronic liver disease or exogenous administration. Other predisposing risk factors include prior chest radiation therapy.

Male breast cancer may be the initial presentation of a *BRCA2* gene carrier family; 85% of these tumours are hormone receptor positive. Prognosis is similar to female breast cancer stage for stage; therefore the management is also similar. Initial approach consists of modified radical mastectomy and axillary node dissection, followed by adjuvant therapies similar to women.

Chemoprevention

In the two largest trials of tamoxifen for primary prevention, tamoxifen was associated with a statistically significant decrease in the risk of ER-positive invasive breast cancer and DCIS, but had no influence on the incidence of ER-negative breast cancer. No study has demonstrated an improvement in overall or breast-cancer-related mortality and tamoxifen is associated with certain serious adverse events. There is an increased risk of endometrial cancer (relative risk 2.4) and thromboembolic events (relative risk 1.9). While the American Society of Clinical Oncology currently suggests consideration of tamoxifen usage in high-risk women, they caution patients to the potential toxicities.

Carcinoma in situ and early breast cancer

- A multi-modality approach to early breast cancer is imperative.
- Breast-conserving techniques are possible in many patients.
- Patients with ER-positive cancers derive most benefit from hormonal therapy.
- Adjuvant chemotherapy is recommended in triple negative patients (ER/PR/HER2neu).

Locally advanced breast cancer (LABC) and inflammatory breast cancer (IBC)

Locally advanced breast cancer constitutes a wide variety of clinical presentations including: large tumours (>5 cm), extensive regional lymph node involvement, direct involvement of the skin or underlying chest wall, tumours considered inoperable but without distant metastasis, and inflammatory breast cancer. With the advent of breast screening programmes less than 5% of breast cancers are stage III. However, in medically under-served areas, locally advanced breast cancers represents 30–50% of breast cancer patients.

Inflammatory breast cancer (IBC) is an aggressive manifestation of locally advanced breast cancer. Its clinical and biological features are characteristic of a rapidly proliferating disease with angio-invasive elements. It represents 1–6% of all malignant breast cancers. The name itself is a misnomer, as the appearances are due to tumour cell invasion of dermal lymphatics, not infiltration of inflammatory cells.

Clinical presentation

Careful examination of the skin, breasts and locoregional lymph nodes is the initial step in evaluating the patient. Most patients will have evidence of a visible and palpable breast mass. IBC has a characteristic appearance with rapid-onset swelling of the breast with erythema (Fig. 1), oedema involving more than two thirds of the breast, peau d'orange (orange skin appearance) (Fig. 2), tenderness, induration, warmth, and diffuse involvement of the breast. Patients will frequently have nodal disease at presentation. Approximately one third will have metastatic disease.

Pathology

The classic findings of inflammatory breast cancer, as mentioned earlier, are dermal lymphatic invasion by tumour cells. The cancer cells are pleomorphic with a high histological grade, highly atypical mitotic figures and a high intra-tumoral vessel density.

These cancers are generally hormone receptor negative, but about two thirds are HER2neu positive.

Staging

Bilateral mammography, radionuclide bone scan, chest CT and ultrasound of the upper abdomen should be performed to exclude the possibility of metastatic disease (Fig. 3).

Management

The management has changed significantly over the years. The importance of the multidisciplinary approach has been established, as single modality therapy is associated with a poor outcome. Combined modality therapy using induction chemotherapy followed by locoregional therapy (surgery and/or radiotherapy) has become the standard of care.

Neoadjuvant chemotherapy, such as anthracyclines or taxanes, is advised as these are the most effective cytotoxics identified to date. One study demonstrated superior results with the sequence of an anthracycline-containing regimen, such as AC (adriamycin and cyclophosphamide), followed by a taxane (docetaxel or paclitaxel). However, in general,

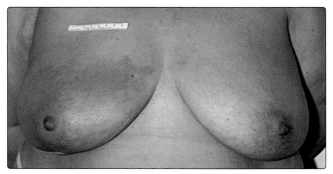

Fig. 1 **Erythematous swollen right breast.** Differential diagnosis is cellulitis versus inflammatory breast cancer.

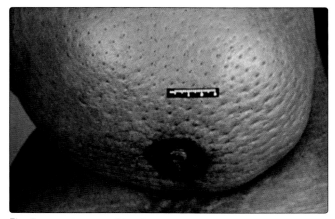

Fig. 2 **Peau d'orange skin effect of breast cancer.**

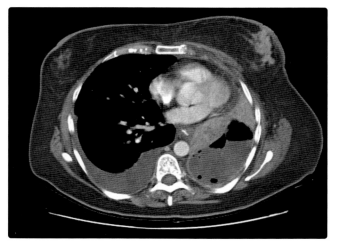

Fig. 3 **CT imaging may identify a breast lesion but is less sensitive and specific.**

cytotoxics used in the adjuvant setting have the potential to be effective in the neoadjuvant setting also. Patients who fail to achieve a response to primary chemotherapy or those with extensive residual disease after chemotherapy have a poor prognosis.

Radiotherapy should be recommended to those patients who fail to respond to neoadjuvant chemotherapy to improve locoregional control.

Table 1 **Disease-free survival (DFS) rates following treatment**		
Therapy for locally advanced breast cancer	**5-year DFS**	**10-year DFS**
Primary radiation	19%	11%
Surgery and radiation	32%	19%
Chemotherapy and radiation	32%	10%
Chemotherapy, surgery and radiation	45%	36%

Hormone therapy should be offered to hormone-receptor-positive patients after completion of systemic chemotherapy and locoregional control (Table 1).

Metastatic breast cancer (MBC)

Despite advances in the management of breast cancer, many patients will develop disease recurrence and 1–5% of patients may have metastatic disease at presentation. The first sites of recurrence or metastases are the chest wall, regional lymph nodes, bone, lung, liver and brain. In women treated for early stage breast cancer the greatest risk of relapse is in the first 5 years; however, over 15% of relapses occur beyond 10 years.

Patients with MBC are unlikely to be cured of their disease. The median survival of all patients with MBC is 2 years; however, 5–10% of patients may survive 5 or more years. A small population of women with metastatic disease have very indolent disease and a long survival.

Management

The focus of therapy is two-fold: prolongation of survival and improvement in quality of life. The improvement in survival may be modest; however, significant improvements in quality of life may be achieved. The aims are to achieve a reduction in disease-related symptoms without excessive treatment-related toxicity.

Management plans should examine both local and systemic treatment options. If a patient has a single site of disease recurrence, local therapy such as resection, radiofrequency ablation or radiotherapy should be employed initially as some patients may be optimally managed with little toxicity until their disease progresses further. The type of systemic therapy depends on performance status of the patient, the progression rate, the extent of the disease, and patient preferences.

Endocrine therapy

Patients with slowly progressive disease, no visceral involvement and minimal symptoms may be best served by a trial of hormonal therapy, even if the tumour has low ER expression. The response rate is lower in ER-poor tumours but never absent.

Premenopausal women could be treated with tamoxifen or ovarian ablation/suppression (oophorectomy, ovarian radio-ablation or drug induced with LHRH agonists). Combined tamoxifen plus an LHRH agonist has a higher response rate and longer time to progression.

Postmenopausal women should be given selective aromatase inhibitors (anastrozole, letrozole or exemestane). There are slightly higher response rates with aromatase inhibitors (AI) than with tamoxifen. However, there does not appear to be any clear advantage of one AI over another. For patients who progress after an AI, tamoxifen should be tried if tamoxifen naïve. Third-line endocrine therapies include fulvestrant, megrestrol acetate or estradiol.

Chemotherapy

For symptomatic patients with rapidly progressive disease, visceral involvement, and a low likelihood of response to hormones or demonstrated hormone refractoriness, chemotherapy is most likely to provide an improvement in quality of life. About two thirds of patients will have some response to chemotherapy, the duration of response lasting between 8 and 12 months. Single agent regimens demonstrate responses of 30%, while combination therapies may have greater responses with potentially greater toxicities. Agents such as anthracyclines (doxorubicin, epirubicin), taxanes (docetaxel, paclitaxel), cyclophosphamide, methotrexate, 5-fluorouracil, vinorelbine and mitomycin C have all shown activity. The optimal duration of therapy has not been established in therapy-responding patients.

Trastuzumab (Herceptin) is appropriate in the management of HER2neu-positive breast cancer. It may be administered as a single agent or in combination with chemotherapy. Superior results have been demonstrated with combination use. At the time of progression, trastuzumab may be combined with a different non-anthracycline agent.

Combination of chemotherapy and hormone therapy should theoretically be better, but some preclinical models suggest that certain combinations may be antagonistic. A meta-analysis of randomised trials detected no survival advantage. High dose chemotherapy with stem cell support has no role in the current management of MBC.

> **Locally advanced breast cancer and inflammatory breast cancer**
>
> - Inflammatory breast cancer is a rapidly progressive cancer with high risk for metastatic spread.
> - 1–5% of women present with metastatic disease despite medical advances.
> - Median survival is 2 years with metastatic breast cancer.
> - The introduction of trastuzumab has improved response rates and survival in HER2neu over-expressing metastatic breast cancer.

Lung cancer

Bronchial carcinoma refers to two distinct clinical entities – small cell and non-small cell carcinoma. Although these conditions have much in common, with broadly similar presenting symptoms, diagnostic procedures and staging systems, their biological behaviour is distinct and this is reflected in their therapeutic management.

Epidemiology
Approximately 37 000 people are diagnosed with lung cancer in the UK annually. Although accounting for 14% of all cancers diagnosed, lung cancer causes 22% of all cancer deaths – it is the commonest cause of cancer death in men and roughly equals the number of breast cancer deaths in women. Older age and lower socio-economic class are significant risk factors.

Aetiology
Tobacco is the commonest cause of lung cancer. Exposure to ionising radiation, asbestos, silica and air pollution are also recognised causative agents.

Smoking
A causative link between lung cancer and smoking was identified in the 1950s. It is currently estimated that >80% of lung cancers in the United Kingdom are caused by smoking. The magnitude of cancer risk increases with the number of cigarettes smoked per day and the number of years spent smoking. Smoking unfiltered cigarettes also increases the risk. Smoking history should be recorded in pack years, with 20 cigarettes per day for one year being equivalent to one pack year.

Carcinogenesis occurs over a period of several decades; therefore the incidence of lung cancer at any time point is reflective of smoking habits in the previous 10 to 20 years. The increasing number of women smoking in the past two decades is reflected in an increased number of deaths from lung cancer.

Cessation of smoking is a valuable public health measure both in terms of cancer risk and benign cardiovascular and respiratory conditions. Lung cancer risk begins to fall 5 years after quitting. The younger a person stops smoking the better, although stopping at any age may be beneficial. National media campaigns promoting the cessation of smoking have met with success rates of 5–10% in many countries.

Pathology
The WHO classification defines five pathological types: small cell (25%), squamous cell (30%), adenocarcinoma (40%), large cell and mixed. Small cell lung carcinoma is frequently characterised by the production of neuroendocrine markers such as chromogranin A and neuron-specific enolase (NSE).

History and examination
Fifteen per cent of patients are asymptomatic at the time of presentation with an incidental finding of a mass on chest X-ray (Fig. 1) precipitating investigation. Non-specific symptoms such as fatigue, malaise, anorexia and weight loss often predominate in the symptomatic patient. Specific symptoms may include haemoptysis, cough, chest pain, hoarseness and dysphagia. A primary lung tumour or enlarged mediastinal nodes may obstruct the airway, predisposing the patient to recurrent or unresolving pneumonia and producing shortness of breath.

Obstruction of the superior vena cava produces a specific syndrome, discussed on page 94. Pancoast's tumours occur in the apex of the lung. They may produce Horner's syndrome (ptosis, myosis and anhidrosis) due to infiltration of the cervical sympathetic chain. Advanced disease typically involves the bone, liver, brain and adrenal glands. Skin deposits may also be seen. Lung cancer is also associated with paraneoplastic syndromes, discussed on page 110.

Clinical signs which should be sought on examination are listed in Box 1. General examination of the patient is critical, allowing assessment of co-morbid conditions common in smokers and an estimate of the patient's fitness for potential treatment modalities.

Diagnosis and staging
Laboratory, radiographic and invasive tests which may be used in the work-up of a suspected lung cancer patient are listed in Table 1. The best method of obtaining a histological diagnosis depends on the location of the tumour. Aspiration of pleural fluid will provide a positive diagnosis on cytology in >50% of cases. Lesions within the bronchi are amenable to biopsy at bronchoscopy. Lesions outside the main bronchi or in the periphery of the lung are usually accessible with a needle inserted through the rib cage. The procedure is called percutaneous transthoracic needle biopsy and is

Box 1 Clinical signs
- Obvious weight loss/cachexia
- Pallor
- Clubbing
- Nicotine staining of the fingers
- Lymphadenopathy – axillary, supraclavicular, cervical
- Collapse/consolidation/effusion in the lung
- Hepatomegaly
- Performance status should be assessed

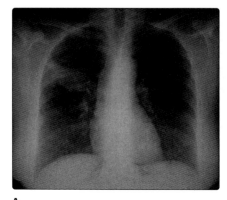

A

B

Fig. 1 **Chest radiograph and corresponding CT scan in a patient with lung cancer.**

Table 1 Work-up of the lung cancer patient

Test	Potential findings
Laboratory tests:	
Full blood count	Anaemia, pancytopenia
Urea and electrolytes	Hyponatraemia, decreased urea in the presence of SIADH
Liver blood tests	Elevated liver enzymes, hypoalbuminaemia
Bone profile	Hypercalcaemia, raised alkaline phosphatase
Lactate dehydrogenase	Raised
Radiology:	
Chest radiograph	Mass lesion, widened mediastinum, pleural effusion, collapse, consolidation, rib erosion
CT scan of thorax/upper abdomen	Definition of extent of primary, presence of enlarged lymph nodes, liver and adrenal metastases
PET scan	Areas of uptake consistent with disease
Isotope bone scan	Areas of uptake consistent with bone metastases
CT brain	Multiple enhancing lesions consistent with brain metastases
MRI	Useful for imaging Pancoast's tumours, brain metastases and bone metastases
Invasive tests:	
Pleural fluid aspiration and cytology	
Sputum cytology	
Bronchoscopy + biopsy, ± lavage	
Percutaneous transthoracic needle biopsy	Histological confirmation of malignancy
Transbronchial biopsy	
Mediastinoscopy	
Bone marrow biopsy	Bone marrow involvement in small cell lung cancer

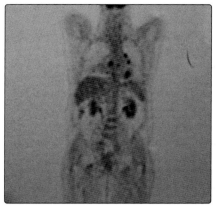

Fig. 2 **PET image showing metastatic disease in mediastinal lymph nodes.** The lower left hotspot reflects normal uptake in the heart. Normal uptake is also seen in the kidneys.

performed under the guidance of CT scan. Transbronchial biopsy implies accessing tumours outside the bronchus by inserting a needle through the bronchial wall. This is associated with a 10% risk of pneumothorax and has largely been superseded by the percutaneous method.

Mediastinoscopy may be undertaken to pathologically stage enlarged mediastinal lymph nodes prior to surgical resection. Pathological confirmation of contralateral mediastinal lymph node involvement will usually render the patient inoperable.

PET scanning has a superior ability to accurately detect active disease in the mediastinum (Fig. 2) and at all distant sites except the brain. This technical advance has translated into a clinical benefit with reduced numbers of unnecessary thoracotomies.

Stage of disease is documented according to the TNM system as shown in Table 2. In clinical practice this system is less useful for small cell lung cancer, which is usually categorised as limited or extensive stage as described in the chapter on small cell lung cancer.

Table 2 Staging for lung cancer

Primary tumour (T)

TX	Primary tumour cannot be assessed, or tumour proven by the presence of malignant cells in sputum or bronchial washings but not visualised by imaging or bronchoscopy
T0	No evidence of primary tumour
Tis	Carcinoma in situ
T1	Tumour 3 cm or less in greatest dimension, surrounded by lung or visceral pleura, without bronchoscopic evidence of invasion more proximal than the lobar bronchus (i.e. not in the main bronchus)
T2	Tumour with any of the following features of size or extent: More than 3 cm in greatest dimension Involves main bronchus, 2 cm or more distal to the carina Invades the visceral pleura Associated with atelectasis or obstructive pneumonitis that extends to the hilar region but does not involve the entire lung
T3	Tumour of any size that directly invades any of the following: chest wall (including superior sulcus tumours), diaphragm, mediastinal pleura, parietal pericardium; or tumour in the main bronchus less than 2 cm distal to the carina, but without involvement of the carina; or associated atelectasis or obstructive pneumonitis of the entire lung
T4	Tumour of any size that invades any of the following: mediastinum, heart, great vessels, trachea, oesophagus, vertebral body, carina; or separate tumour nodules in the same lobe; or tumour with malignant pleural effusion

Regional lymph nodes (N)

NX	Regional lymph nodes cannot be assessed
N0	No regional lymph node metastasis
N1	Metastasis to ipsilateral peribronchial and/or ipsilateral hilar lymph nodes, and intrapulmonary nodes including involvement by direct extension of the primary tumour
N2	Metastasis to ipsilateral mediastinal and/or subcarinal lymph node(s)
N3	Metastasis to contralateral mediastinal, contralateral hilar, ipsilateral or contralateral scalene, or supraclavicular lymph node(s)

Distant metastasis (M)

MX	Distant metastasis cannot be assessed
M0	No distant metastasis
M1	Distant metastasis

Used with the permission of the American Joint Committee on Cancer (AJCC), Chicago, Illinois. The original source for this material is the *AJCC Cancer Staging Manual*, Sixth Edition (2002) published by Springer-New York, www.springeronline.com.

Lung cancer

- Lung cancer is the commonest cause of cancer death.
- Smoking is the major causative factor.
- The commonest type of lung cancer is non-small cell lung cancer, with adenocarcinoma and squamous cell carcinoma accounting for most cases.
- Non-small cell lung cancer is staged using the TNM system.
- Small cell lung cancer is usually staged as limited or extensive.

Non-small cell lung cancer

Non-small cell lung cancer is associated with a poor prognosis. The majority of patients present with advanced disease which is not amenable to curative surgery. Combined treatment with radiotherapy and chemotherapy is beneficial for some patients but the overall outcome remains poor; 5-year survival is <10% and only one quarter of patients survive for one year or more.

Staging

The TNM staging system as described on page 23 is also expressed in stage groupings from I to IV, with distinct variations in prognosis as shown in Table 1. A patient who is considered suitable for surgery or radical radiotherapy after a CT scan should go on to have a PET scan to assess the nodes in the mediastinum. These nodes are the initial site of spread in non-small cell lung cancer as illustrated in Fig. 1.

If the PET scan is negative, indicating that the nodes are not involved, the patient may proceed to surgery or radiotherapy. If the PET scan is positive, showing involvement of the ipsilateral mediastinal nodes (N1), the patient may still proceed to surgery. If there is more extensive lymph node involvement (N2 or N3) on the PET scan, the cancer may be inoperable. A biopsy of these nodes will clarify the stage before proceeding to radical surgery or radiotherapy.

Management

Stages I and II

Surgery

Complete surgical resection provides the patient with the best chance of long-term survival. The type of surgical procedure performed depends on the size of the primary tumour, its precise anatomical location and proximity to mediastinal structures. In all cases the aim of successful surgery is to remove the cancer with clear margins.

- Wedge resection – small section of lung removed, suitable for small primary tumours in the periphery of the lung.
- Lobectomy – removal of a single lobe. This is the most commonly performed operation for lung cancer.
- Pneumonectomy – removal of the entire lung. Preoperative assessment of lung function is critical.
- Sleeve resection – indicated for centrally placed tumours. May allow patient to avoid pneumonectomy.

All patients undergoing surgical resection of a lung tumour should have sampling of the lymph nodes to establish the pathological stage of disease.

Medically inoperable patients

Many patients presenting with lung cancer have significant co-morbid cardiovascular and respiratory illness. A baseline assessment of cardiac and lung function is required prior to any intervention. All patients should have pulmonary function tests performed to assess fitness for surgery or radical radiotherapy. An FEV1 (forced expiratory volume in 1 second) of 1 L is often used as an indicator of the feasibility of extensive resection. Patients considered at substantial risk of life-threatening complications after surgery may be offered radical radiotherapy as an alternative.

Adjuvant chemotherapy

Patients who have had a complete resection of stage IB or stage II cancer can be offered adjuvant chemotherapy. Cisplatin- or carboplatin-based treatment has been shown to improve survival in meta-analyses in recent years.

Adjuvant radiotherapy

A patient with a positive resection margin may be considered for postoperative radiotherapy to improve local control. Radiotherapy and chemotherapy should not be given concurrently in this setting because

Table 1 Stage grouping and prognosis for non-small cell lung cancer			
Stage		**TNM characteristics**	**Approximate 5-year survival**
I	IA	T1N0	60–80%
	IB	T2N0	
II	IIA	T1N1	50%
	IIB	T2N1	
		T3N0	
III	IIIA	T1/2N2	10–25%
		T3N1/2	
	IIIB	Any T, N3	
		T4, any N	
IV		Any T, any N, M1	<5%

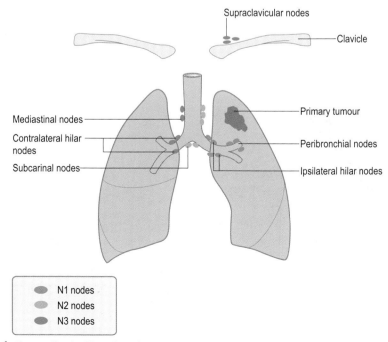

Fig. 1 **The mediastinal lymph nodes.**

the combination is associated with increased toxicity and has not been tested extensively in the postoperative patient group.

Stage III

Stage III disease includes a heterogeneous group of patients; some are suitable for radical surgical procedures but many are elderly with inoperable disease, suitable for palliative treatment. The optimal treatment may be a matter of discussion, best managed at a multidisciplinary team meeting.

Resectable stage III disease

Surgery

Carefully selected patients with stage III disease may be suitable for radical resection and should be offered surgery. In general, bulky N2 nodal disease is considered a contraindication to surgery. T4 primary tumours are usually unresectable; however, in the case of involvement of the chest wall, complete resection of the tumour with the affected portion of the chest wall may be attempted. Individual cases should be assessed by a multi-disciplinary team after full work-up.

Adjuvant chemotherapy and radiotherapy

Adjuvant chemotherapy and radiotherapy may be offered depending on the surgical and pathological findings.

Unresectable stage III disease

Radical chemoradiotherapy

Chemoradiotherapy is indicated when disease is not amenable to surgery. The combination of chemotherapy and radiotherapy may be given sequentially or concurrently. Concurrent treatment may be more effective but results in increased toxicity. Further studies are required to provide robust evidence of the superiority of concurrent treatment. Chemotherapy regimens combining a platinum agent such as carboplatin or cisplatin with a second agent such as paclitaxel or gemcitabine are commonly used.

Stage IV

Palliative treatment should be tailored to meet the needs of the individual patient. Chemotherapy in addition to supportive care is beneficial in patients with a good performance status.

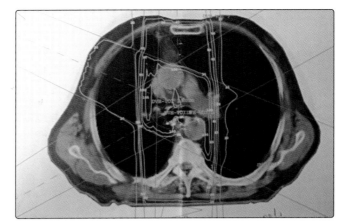

Fig. 2 **CT plan for lung tumour.** The green lines represent radiation beams, the blue are lines of equal dose – isodose lines, as calculated by the radiotherapy planning system.

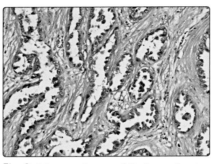

Fig. 3 **Adenocarcinoma of the lung.** Courtesy of Dr David Delaney.

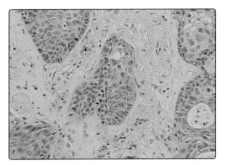

Fig. 4 **Squamous cell carcinoma of the lung.** Courtesy of Dr David Delaney.

Radiotherapy

Radiotherapy treatment techniques for lung cancer have advanced significantly with the advent of CT-based planning. This technique allows precise definition of the area to be treated on CT slices through the thorax and provides accurate information regarding the percentage of normal tissue exposed to the radiation dose.

The clinical target volume will include the primary tumour and the involved lymph nodes with a suitable margin to allow for microscopic extension of disease. This target volume is outlined on CT slices as shown in Fig. 2. Using conventional fractionation, a total dose of 66 Gy at 2 Gy per fraction over $6^{1}/_{2}$ weeks may be delivered, keeping the dose to normal tissues within safe limits.

Continuous hyperfractionated accelerated radiotherapy (CHART)

CHART refers to treatment given in smaller, more numerous fractions (hyperfractionation) over a shorter time period (acceleration), e.g. 54 Gy delivered at 1.5 Gy per fraction over 12 days with three fractions given each day. Randomised trials have shown a significant survival benefit for this protocol. However, widespread implementation is problematic due to the practical demands on resources. A modified version of CHART, which does not involve treatment at the weekends, has been used as an alternative.

Non-small cell lung cancer

- Management guidelines are based on the stage of disease at presentation.

- Radical resection should be offered if possible – complete resection provides the best chance of long-term survival.

- Adjuvant chemotherapy should be offered to patients with completely resected disease.

- Adjuvant radiotherapy increases local control in incompletely resected disease.

- Chemoradiotherapy should be offered to patients with unresectable disease.

- Medically inoperable patients should be considered for radiotherapy.

- The 5-year survival varies from <5% to 80% depending on the stage of disease.

Small cell lung cancer

Introduction

Small cell lung cancer is a systemic disease – up to 70% of patients have distant metastases at the time of presentation. Most patients develop metastatic disease during the course of their illness. For this reason, standard treatment relies on chemotherapy with or without the addition of radiotherapy. There is little role for surgery, which is indicated only in patients with very limited disease within the chest. Patients with small cell lung cancer should be encouraged to participate in clinical trials as part of ongoing efforts to improve prognosis.

Staging

The TNM staging system described in Table 2 on page 23 also applies to small cell lung cancer. However, in clinical practice a simpler staging system is commonly used. According to this system, patients are classified as having limited or extensive stage disease:

- Limited stage disease is confined to one side of the chest with no evidence of metastatic disease. It may alternatively be defined as disease which can be incorporated in a radiotherapy treatment field. The latter definition is a pragmatic one as the standard treatment for limited stage disease includes radiotherapy.
- Extensive disease includes patients with distant metastases outside the ipsilateral hemithorax.

Specific staging investigations used for lung cancer are described on page 23. The most important prognostic factors as listed below should be documented prior to treatment.

Features associated with a better prognosis include:

- limited stage disease
- younger age
- better performance status
- normal lactate dehydrogenase level
- normal sodium level
- normal albumin level.

Management

Limited stage disease

Combined treatment with chemotherapy and radiotherapy is the standard of care. Chemotherapy is the key component of treatment – radiotherapy alone does not alter long-term outcome. Chemotherapy is given first by convention. This allows an estimation of the degree of responsiveness of the disease to chemotherapy, a factor which may influence the decision to give further chemotherapy when disease recurs. Additionally, in practical terms, most oncology services find it easier to start chemotherapy quickly rather than radiotherapy.

The optimal timing of treatment, either concurrent or sequential, is the subject of discussion. There is evidence from randomised trials and meta-analyses that commencing radiotherapy early in the course of chemotherapy improves overall survival compared to later introduction of radiotherapy. However, the combined schedule is associated with an increase in toxicity which may make it an unsuitable treatment option for some patients.

Chemotherapy

A combination of a platinum drug (cisplatin or carboplatin) with etoposide is the most commonly used treatment regimen. This is favoured in the setting of combined treatment with radiotherapy as it is associated with less toxicity. Other regimens in common use are listed in Table 1. Four to six cycles of chemotherapy are given. Longer schedules or the use of maintenance chemotherapy are not beneficial.

Small cell lung cancer is very sensitive to chemotherapy. Up to 90% of patients with limited stage disease respond to chemotherapy; approximately half of these will be complete responses. The response seen on CT scan after four cycles of chemotherapy is illustrated in Fig. 1. Unfortunately, disease recurrence is the norm, resulting in poor long-term survival in spite of initial sensitivity to treatment.

Radiotherapy

Thoracic radiotherapy reduces the risk of recurrence and increases long-term survival when given with chemotherapy. Areas of gross disease only are included within the treatment field. Prophylactic treatment of uninvolved nodal areas is not necessary as it does not improve outcome and significantly increases toxicity. The oncologist may choose to include areas of gross disease at presentation or, in patients receiving sequential treatment, only the areas of gross disease remaining after response to chemotherapy. A typical radiotherapy treatment schedule is 50 Gy delivered in 2 Gy fractions, given once daily over 5 weeks.

Extensive stage disease

Combination chemotherapy as described for limited stage disease is the treatment of choice for patients with a reasonable performance status. Patients who are not fit for chemotherapy should be given supportive care and referred to their local palliative care service. Thirty to forty per cent of patients achieve a response to chemotherapy, a minority of these achieving a complete response.

Prophylactic cranial irradiation

Brain metastases are extremely common in small cell lung cancer. Even patients who have a complete response or a good partial response to combined modality treatment will go on to develop brain metastases in approximately half the cases. This event is associated with significant morbidity and mortality, with profound effects on the well-being of both patient and family.

Prophylactic irradiation of the whole brain was introduced with a view to reducing the incidence of brain metastases and has been proven to do so. A meta-analysis has also shown that prophylactic irradiation also improves long-term survival. At present it is recommended that patients with limited stage disease who achieve a

Table 1 **Combination chemotherapy for small cell lung cancer**	
Regimen	**Drugs**
EP	Cisplatin
	Etoposide
ICE	Ifosfamide
	Carboplatin
	Etoposide
CAV	Cyclophosphamide
	Doxorubicin (Adriamycin)
	Vincristine
CAE	Cyclophosphamide
	Doxorubicin (Adriamycin)
	Etoposide

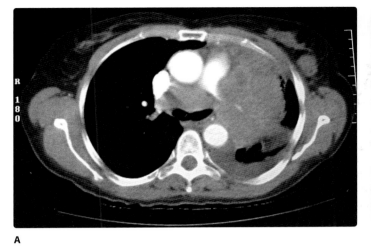

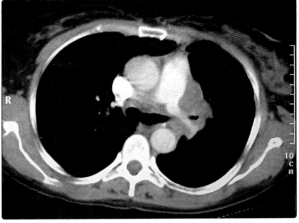

A   B

Fig. 1 **CT scan before (A) and after (B) chemotherapy for small cell lung cancer.**

good partial response or complete response to combined modality treatment should be offered prophylactic cranial irradiation. Patients with extensive stage disease who achieve a complete response at sites of distant metastases should also be considered for treatment.

Whole cranial irradiation is associated with potential long-term effects on cognitive function. The analysis of cognitive impairment in patients with small cell lung cancer has been confounded by the fact that the cancer itself may be associated with neurocognitive defects. Chemotherapy drugs, their doses and timing also impact on the potential effect of radiation. However, it is now generally accepted that the benefits of cranial irradiation in these patients outweigh the risks of potential long-term cognitive effects.

Doses in the region of 30 Gy are administered. In order to minimise toxicity, daily fractions should not exceed 2–2.5 Gy and cranial irradiation

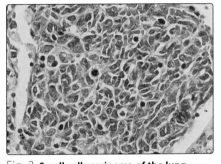

Fig. 2 **Small cell carcinoma of the lung (×40).** Courtesy of Dr David Delaney.

should not be administered concurrently with chemotherapy.

Prognosis

Small cell lung cancer is associated with extremely limited survival times in untreated patients, of the order of 4 months and 2 months for limited stage and extensive stage disease, respectively. Treatment has a significant impact on median survival, which increases to approximately 18 months in limited stage disease and 9 months in extensive stage disease.

Small cell lung cancer

- Small cell lung cancer is staged as limited or extensive disease.
- Chemotherapy and thoracic radiotherapy is the standard treatment for limited stage disease.
- Prophylactic cranial irradiation reduces the incidence of brain metastases and prolongs survival in certain groups of patients.
- The approximate median survival for limited stage disease is 4 months if untreated and 18 months if treated.
- The approximate median survival for extensive stage disease is 2 months if untreated and 9 months if treated.

Mesothelioma

This uncommon cancer arises from mesothelial cells which are present in the serosal lining of the pleura, pericardium and peritoneal cavities. There are fewer than 1500 new cases of mesothelioma diagnosed each year. There is a male to female predominance, with a male to female ratio of 5 to 1. The median overall survival is 11 months after diagnosis.

Aetiology

Eighty per cent of patients have a history of asbestos exposure. Mesothelioma has a peak incidence 35–45 years after asbestos exposure. Asbestos was widely used in insulation up to the 1980s. Box 1 outlines occupations at greatest risk of exposure. Although all types of asbestos can cause mesothelioma, the most carcinogenic is crocidolite (Box 2). Asbestos has carcinogenic effects via different mechanisms (Box 3). Smoking acts synergistically with asbestos to increase the risk of developing mesothelioma.

Chronic pleurisy, radiation and Thorotrast (contrast medium) exposure are associated with increased risk. Simian virus 40 may also have an oncogenic role.

Clinical presentation

Most patients present in their sixth or seventh decade with increasing dyspnoea and chest pain. However, peritoneal mesothelioma generally presents with increasing abdominal girth caused by ascites. Constitutional symptoms which include anorexia, weight loss, fatigue and night sweats are common.

Pathology

Three histological variants have been described: epithelial, sarcomatoid and mixed. The epithelial variant occurs in over 60% of cases and is associated with the best prognosis. Although a comprehensive immunohistochemical pattern should definitively diagnose mesothelioma, electron microscopy remains the gold standard.

Diagnosis and staging

Pleural effusion, which has a predilection for the right side, is the most common X-ray finding (Fig. 1). Less than 5% of cases will have bilateral disease. CT is required to visualise pleural thickening and determines anatomical involvement for staging (Figs 2 and 3). While imaging is used to stage patients, more definitive staging is often only possible at the time of surgery.

Box 1 Occupations at risk of asbestos exposure

- Thermal insulation engineers
- Asbestos manufacturing workers
- Shipyard workers
- Builders
- Plumbers
- Electricians
- Gas fitters
- Carpenters

Box 2 Asbestos subtypes

- Chrysotile (white)
- Amosite (brown)
- Crocidolite (blue)
- Tremolite
- Actinolite
- Anthophyllite

Box 3 Mechanism of carcinogenesis

- Direct chromosomal toxicity
- DNA strand breaks
- Free radical induced deletions
- Production of inflammatory cytokines

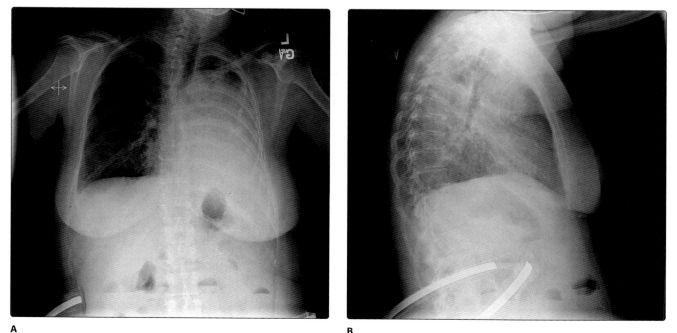

A   B

Fig. 1 **Chest X-ray demonstrating pleural effusion.** Anteroposterior film (A) shows opacification of the left lung, and on lateral view (B) the left hemidiaphragm is not seen.

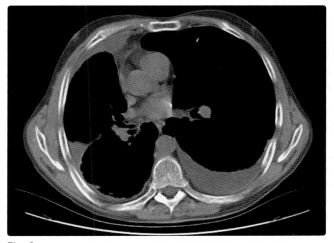

Fig. 2 **CT demonstrating complicated bilateral effusions.** The right side is loculated as a result of pleural thickening and fibrosis.

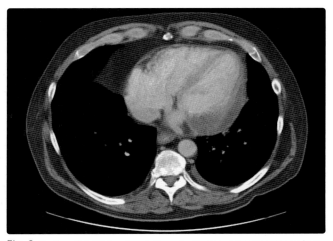

Fig. 3 **Pericardial thickening, left posterior heart border, secondary to mesothelioma.**

PET scan, while more sensitive than CT for finding extrathoracic disease, has limited sensitivity for local staging and determining potential for resection.

Adequate tissue is required to differentiate between mesothelioma and lung cancer. There is a risk of seeding with closed lung biopsy.

Management
The only curative therapy is complete surgical resection; however, this is rarely possible. Extrapleural pneumonectomy involves complete removal of the ipsilateral lung along with the parietal and visceral pleura, pericardium with portions of the phrenic nerve, and the majority of the hemidiaphragm. This procedure is technically difficult, with a 5% postoperative mortality.

Surgical palliative approaches include pleurodesis or pleurectomy (decortication). Decortication may be more successful for palliation of symptoms, but it does not result in survival benefit and is associated with morbidity. Certain factors with prognostic importance are outlined in Table 1.

Radiation is sometimes considered as an adjuvant therapy primarily to prevent chest wall recurrences. Chemotherapy may be used as an adjunct or in the palliative setting. Agents with some activity include doxorubicin, platinum agents and pemetrexed. Although single agents have some response, at present the most effective regimen consists of pemetrexed and a platinum compound.

Asbestos exposure compensation
People suffering from asbestos-induced diseases can usually take legal action against employers who exposed them to dangerous quantities of asbestos. They can also apply to the Benefits Agency for industrial injuries benefit if they suffer

Table 1 **Prognostic factors**	
Good prognosis	**Poor prognosis**
Epithelial histology	Sarcomatoid histology
Stage I disease	Advanced stage disease
Age <65 years	Age >65 years
Good performance status (WHO score 0–1)	Poor performance status
	Fever of unknown origin
	Anaemia
	Leucocytosis

from various asbestos-related conditions known as 'prescribed diseases' which includes asbestosis, bilateral diffuse pleural thickening, lung cancer accompanied by one of the first two conditions, and mesothelioma. Pleural plaques alone are not recognised for compensation by the Benefits Agency. Advice can be sought from either from the British Lung Foundation helpline on 08458 50 50 20, or local Citizens Advice Bureau.

> **Mesothelioma**
>
> - Mesothelioma is an unusual cancer, with over 80% of patients having a history of asbestos exposure.
> - A lag period of 30–40 years occurs before development of cancer.
> - The only curative option is surgical resection, but this is rarely possible.
> - The new antifolate agent pemetrexed has shown some promise.
> - Compensation is possible for asbestos-related lung damage.

Colorectal cancer

Introduction

Colorectal cancer is the third most commonly diagnosed cancer in both men and women in the UK. It is also the third most common cause of cancer death. Survival has steadily improved over the past 20 years with improved treatment and an enhanced understanding of the natural history of the disease.

Aetiology

Both sporadic and hereditary forms of colorectal cancer occur. Causative factors related to sporadic colorectal cancer are listed in Box 1. Around 10–15% of cases may be accounted for by an inherited genetic predisposition, the commonest conditions being hereditary non-polyposis colorectal cancer (HNPCC) and familial adenomatous polyposis (FAP).

Pathology

Most colorectal cancers arise in the sigmoid colon and rectum. The gross appearance is variable and may be polypoid, infiltrative or ulcerative. The majority are adenocarcinomas arising in a pre-existing adenoma. An adenoma is a benign lesion with malignant potential.

The progression from normal mucosa to adenoma to adenocarcinoma is now known in some detail. The accumulation of genetic defects in this sequence takes time, which is one of the reasons why sporadic cases are increasingly common with age, typically presenting at >50 years of age. Familial conditions often present much earlier.

Colorectal cancers may spread via the lymphatic or haematogenous route or across the peritoneal cavity. The pathologist is largely responsible for determining the stage on the basis of surgical specimens.

History and examination

Presenting symptoms depend on the location of the primary cancer within the bowel (Fig. 1). Non-specific symptoms include weight loss, malaise and fatigue. Acute presentation with obstruction or perforation is not uncommon.

Rectal cancer is usually diagnosed on digital rectal examination. Examination of the abdomen may reveal abdominal mass, hepatomegaly or inguinal nodes. Respiratory examination may reveal signs of lung metastases. Performance status should also be evaluated.

Investigations

- *Colonoscopy* allows visualisation of tumour extent and biopsy to confirm the diagnosis. Full colonoscopy is important as synchronous tumours occur.
- *Laboratory tests* – routine investigations include full blood count, renal and liver function tests. Carcinoembryonic antigen (CEA) and carbohydrate antigen (CA) 19–9 are increased in the presence of colorectal cancer. These tumour markers are non-specific, but they can be used to assess response to treatment.
- *Radiology* – the extent of the tumour within the abdomen/pelvis and the presence of distant metastases is often assessed with CT scan. MRI may detect liver metastases missed on CT scanning, which may alter management in some patients. PET scans are useful in specific situations. Abdominal ultrasound and chest X-ray may also be used as staging investigations. A double contrast barium enema may be diagnostic when full colonoscopy is not possible.

Staging

Several staging systems have been used for colorectal cancer, all based on similar prognostic factors: depth of invasion of primary tumour, extent of nodal involvement and presence of distant metastases. This was originally described in the Dukes staging system and subsequently modified by Astler and Coller. The current staging system is illustrated in Table 1.

Management

Surgery

Surgery is the curative treatment in colorectal cancer. Most polyps can be safely removed endoscopically. Curative surgery of invasive cancers requires radical resection of the tumour with a sufficient margin and lymphadenectomy to remove the draining lymph nodes. The procedure performed depends on the location of the primary tumour within the bowel. Rectal tumours may require abdominoperineal resection and

---

Box 1 Aetiology of colorectal cancer

Risk factors
- Increasing age
- Familial predisposition
- Ulcerative colitis – risk depends on disease extent and duration. Extensive disease for >10 years confers a significantly increased risk
- Diabetes
- Cholecystectomy
- Diet high in red meat content
- Smoking

Protective factors
- Diet high in vegetables and fibre
- Aspirin and other non-steroidal anti-inflammatory drugs

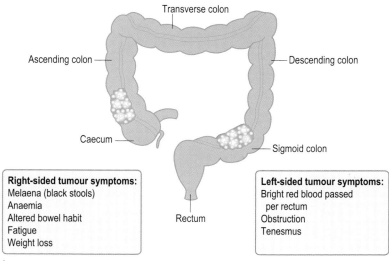

Right-sided tumour symptoms:
Melaena (black stools)
Anaemia
Altered bowel habit
Fatigue
Weight loss

Left-sided tumour symptoms:
Bright red blood passed
    per rectum
Obstruction
Tenesmus

Transverse colon
Ascending colon
Descending colon
Caecum
Sigmoid colon
Rectum

Fig. 1 **Symptoms of colorectal cancer.**

Table 1 **Staging for colorectal cancer**	
Primary tumour (T)	
TX	Primary tumour cannot be assessed
T0	No evidence of primary tumour
Tis	Carcinoma in situ: intraepithelial or invasion of lamina propria
T1	Tumour invades submucosa
T2	Tumour invades muscularis propria
T3	Tumour invades through the muscularis propria into the subserosa, or into non-peritonealised pericolic or perirectal tissues
T4	Tumour directly invades other organs or structures, and/or perforates visceral peritoneum
Regional lymph nodes (N)	
NX	Regional lymph nodes cannot be assessed
N0	No regional lymph node metastasis
N1	Metastasis in 1 to 3 regional lymph nodes
N2	Metastasis in 4 or more regional lymph nodes
Distant metastasis (M)	
MX	Distant metastasis cannot be assessed
M0	No distant metastasis
M1	Distant metastasis

Used with the permission of the American Joint Committee on Cancer (AJCC), Chicago, Illinois. The original source for this material is the *AJCC Cancer Staging Manual*, Sixth Edition (2002) published by Springer-New York, www.springeronline.com.

> ## Box 2 The Amsterdam criteria in the diagnosis of HNPCC
>
> - Involvement of at least two successive generations
> - At least one case diagnosed before the age of 50 years
> - At least three relatives with colorectal cancer, one of whom must be a first degree relative of the other two

permanent colostomy (see p. 14). Total mesorectal excision during resection of rectal cancer has been proven to reduce the risk of local recurrence and is the procedure of choice. More proximal tumours may be treated with anterior resection or hemicolectomy.

Chemotherapy and radiotherapy
Recurrence rates of up to 40% after surgery alone led to the introduction of adjuvant chemotherapy and radiotherapy. There is clear evidence that adjuvant chemotherapy reduces disease recurrence and increases survival in node-positive colorectal cancer. Initially all trials focused on postoperative treatment; however, it now seems likely that neoadjuvant preoperative treatment is superior in the treatment of locally advanced rectal cancer. Adjuvant radiotherapy is indicated in resected node-positive rectal cancer or rectal cancer that has penetrated the full thickness of the bowel wall.

Chemotherapy
The antimetabolite 5-fluorouracil is the most commonly prescribed agent in the treatment of colorectal cancer. It may be administered as a bolus using a number of different schedules or as a continuous infusion through an indwelling catheter using a pump system (Fig. 2). Leucovorin, which potentiates the action of 5-fluorouracil, is usually given concurrently although it may be omitted if the patient is also receiving radiotherapy to avoid an unacceptable increase in side effects. The addition of a new agent, oxaliplatin, to 5-fluorouracil and leucovorin combinations gives

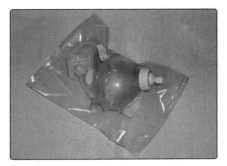

Fig. 2 **Continuous infusion pump.** The pump is connected to an indwelling catheter and carried in a pouch worn by the patient on a belt.

superior results in high-risk node-positive patients.

Treatment of metastatic disease
Palliative treatment should be tailored to the individual patient with intervention depending on symptoms and performance status. Palliative resection of the primary tumour may significantly improve symptoms and avoid obstruction in the future. Patients not fit for surgery may respond to hypofractionated palliative radiotherapy regimens. Patients with a good performance status will benefit from palliative chemotherapy, which can improve quality of life and increase median survival.

Hepatic and pulmonary resection
Resection of hepatic and pulmonary metastases can be associated with long-term survival in carefully selected patients. MRI is preferable for investigation of liver metastases in this setting as it is more likely to pick up additional lesions not seen on CT that may render the patient unsuitable for surgery. Surgery is often followed by further chemotherapy.

HNPCC
The clinical presentation of HNPCC may be indistinguishable from sporadic cases of colorectal carcinoma. Diagnosis requires a high degree of suspicion on the part of the physician and proactive investigation of the family history in all cases. The Amsterdam criteria (Box 2) are applied to make a diagnosis on the basis of family history. Surveillance colonoscopy should be carried out in all affected family members. Treatment is associated with a similar outcome to sporadic cases.

FAP
This condition, unlike HNPCC, is readily apparent on colonoscopy as the bowel is covered in thousands of polyps and progression to cancer is inevitable. Surveillance colonoscopy is of no value as any of the polyps may become cancerous. Prophylactic colectomy performed during the teenage years is recommended to reduce the risk of cancer.

> ## Colorectal cancer
>
> - Colorectal cancer is the third most commonly diagnosed cancer in men and women in the UK and the third commonest cause of cancer death.
> - Most colorectal cancers are adenocarcinomas arising in adenomatous polyps.
> - Surgery is the curative treatment.
>
> - Adjuvant chemotherapy is of proven benefit in node-positive colorectal cancer.
> - Preoperative radiotherapy is of benefit in locally advanced rectal cancer.
> - HNPCC and FAP are the commonest hereditary causes of colorectal cancer.

Gastric cancer

There are over 9000 new cases of gastric cancer per year. It represents the fifth most common cancer in men in the UK. The median age of presentation is in the sixth decade. Only one fifth of patients present with operable disease; overall, the 5-year survival for patients with unresectable disease is <5%.

Aetiology

Chronic *Helicobacter pylori* infection can cause gastritis and chronic inflammation, which are crucial steps in carcinogenesis. Infection has been associated with a six-fold increase in the risk of adenocarcinoma. Large epidemiological studies have identified that certain diets increase the risk of gastric cancer. Dietary nitrates from cured foods and high salt intake are strongly associated with increased risk; increased risk has also been noted with diets low in vegetables, fruits and vitamin A or high in fried food, processed meat and fish. Risk factors for gastric cancer are outlined in Box 1.

Clinical presentation

The common presenting symptoms of gastric cancer are weight loss and abdominal pain. Fig. 1 outlines the most common sites of primary disease. Other presentations include: anaemia secondary to occult blood loss, anorexia, early satiety and dyspepsia. Advanced gastric cancer may present with a pigmented peri-umbilical nodule (Sister Mary Joseph's nodule) or a left supraclavicular lymph node (Virchow's node). Fig. 2 outlines the sites of metastatic disease.

A wide variety of paraneoplastic disorders have been described as the initial presentation of gastric cancer.

Pathology

The majority of gastric cancers are carcinomas, of which over 95% are adenocarcinomas. The signet ring cancer cell is pathognomonic of gastric cancer (Fig. 3). The histological subtypes are outlined in Box 2. Gastric cancer follows a well-developed carcinogenesis model passing through stages of: chronic gastritis, atrophic gastritis, metaplasia, dysplasia to adenocarcinoma. Histologically linitis plastica, the name given to a diffuse infiltrative process often involving the entire gastric mucosa, has a characteristic 'leather bottle' appearance on barium studies.

Other pathologies seen are gastric lymphomas, carcinoid tumours or gastrointestinal stromal tumours (GISTs).

Diagnosis and staging

Although barium studies may identify suspicious lesions, a significant number of false negative studies may occur. Diagnosis is established with upper endoscopy and biopsy; greater diagnostic yield is achieved with multiple biopsies. Tumours of the gastro-oesophageal junction may be difficult to stage appropriately; if more than 50% of the tumour is below the gastro-oesophageal junction it is classified as a gastric cancer. Preoperative clinical staging consists of CT scan of chest and abdomen. However, surgical staging is more accurate (Table 1).

Endoscopic ultrasound may be a useful staging tool in experienced hands. It can determine depth of tumour invasion or lymph node involvement. Laparoscopy should be considered for all good performance status patients with potentially resectable disease.

Box 1 Risk factors

- Dietary
  High salt or nitrates
  Smoked foods
- Smoking
- *Helicobacter pylori* infection
- Radiation exposure
- Prior gastric surgery
- Genetic factors
  HNPCC[a]
  Pernicious anaemia
  Li–Fraumeni syndrome[b]
  Family history of gastric cancer
  Type A blood group

[a]HNPCC (Lynch syndrome) – an autosomal dominant disorder caused by mutations in DNA mismatch repair proteins.
[b]Li–Fraumeni syndrome – a rare autosomal dominant syndrome predisposed to multiple cancers.

Box 2 Gastric carcinoma: histological subtypes

- Adenocarcinoma
- Papillary adenocarcinoma
- Tubular adenocarcinoma
- Mucinous adenocarcinoma
- Signet ring cell carcinoma
- Adenosquamous carcinoma
- Squamous cell carcinoma
- Small cell carcinoma
- Undifferentiated carcinoma

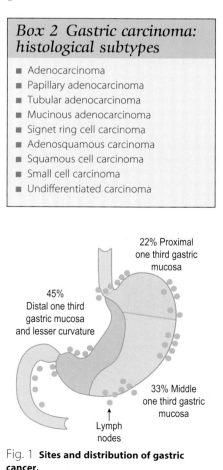

22% Proximal one third gastric mucosa

45% Distal one third gastric mucosa and lesser curvature

33% Middle one third gastric mucosa

Lymph nodes

Fig. 1 **Sites and distribution of gastric cancer.**

Table 1	**TNM staging for gastric cancer**
Tumour	
TX	Cannot be assessed
T0	No evidence of primary tumour
Tis	Carcinoma in situ
T1	Invades lamina propria or submucosa
T2	Invades muscularis propria or subserosa
T3	Invades serosa without invasion of adjacent structures
T4	Invades adjacent structures
Nodes	
NX	Cannot be assessed
N0	No regional lymph nodes involved
N1	1–6 Regional lymph nodes involved
N2	7–15 Regional lymph nodes involved
N3	>15 Regional lymph nodes involved
Metastasis	
MX	Cannot be assessed
M0	No metastasis
M1	Distant metastasis
Stage	
Stage 0	TisN0M0
Stage IA	T1N0M0
Stage IB	T1N1M0
	T2N0M0
Stage II	T1N2M0
	T2N1M0
	T3N0M0
Stage IIIA	T2N2M0
	T3N1M0
	T4N0M0
Stage IIIB	T3N2M0
Stage IV	Any T, N1–3, M0–1

Used with the permission of the American Joint Committee on Cancer (AJCC), Chicago, Illinois. The original source for this material is the *AJCC Cancer Staging Manual*, Sixth edition (2002) published by Springer-New York, www.springeronline.com.

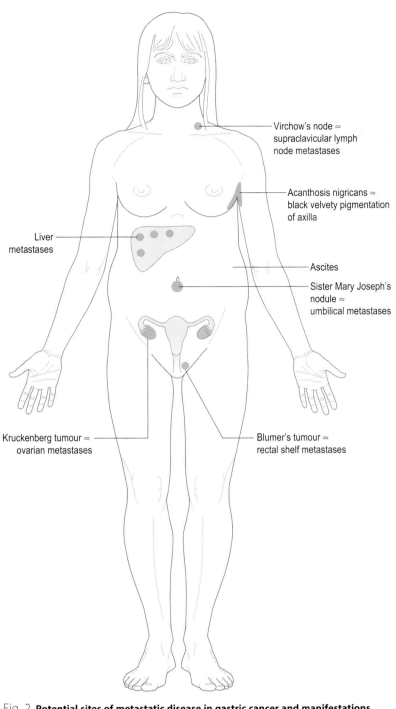

Fig. 2 **Potential sites of metastatic disease in gastric cancer and manifestations.**

Virchow's node ≈ supraclavicular lymph node metastases

Acanthosis nigricans ≈ black velvety pigmentation of axilla

Liver metastases

Ascites

Sister Mary Joseph's nodule ≈ umbilical metastases

Kruckenberg tumour ≈ ovarian metastases

Blumer's tumour ≈ rectal shelf metastases

Table 2 **Survival rates**	
Stage	**5-year survival rate**
Stage 0	>90%
Stage IA	60–80%
Stage IB	50–60%
Stage II	30–50%
Stage IIIA	<20%
Stage IIIB	<10%
Stage IV	<5%

of adjuvant and neoadjuvant chemotherapeutic approaches (Table 2). A UK MRC trial, of over 500 patients, compared surgery alone to combination therapy. Combined chemotherapy and surgical therapy had superior overall survival, with reduced local failure rates and metastatic rates.

Chemotherapy can be useful in the palliative management of advanced gastric cancer, improving quality of life and prolonging survival. A 20% response rate is seen with single agent chemotherapies such as 5-fluorouracil, doxorubicin, platinums, taxanes or irinotecan. Endoscopic laser, radiation or palliative surgery may be of help to minimise symptoms such as bleeding.

Gastric lymphoma

Primary gastric lymphoma is an uncommon disease and accounts for less than 10% of gastric cancers. The majority are of B-cell origin. Pathology varies from well-differentiated superficial mucosal involvement (mucosa-associated lymphatic tissue lymphomas – MALToma) to high-grade large cell lymphomas. There is a strong association with *Helicobacter pylori*; other risk factors include HIV and immunosuppression. While antibiotic therapy may be effective in 60% of cases of MALToma, systemic chemotherapy is needed for management of high-grade lymphomas.

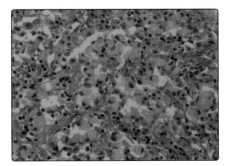

Fig. 3 **Gastric signet ring cell carcinoma.**

The most common metastatic sites are liver, peritoneal surfaces and non-regional lymph nodes. Pulmonary and CNS metastases occur less frequently.

Regional lymph node architecture may be completely replaced by adenocarcinoma; therefore tumour nodules found in the fat adjacent to gastric cancer are considered as positive regional lymph nodes.

Management
Surgical resection is the only potentially curative option. Total gastrectomy is considered for lesions of the upper third while subtotal gastrectomy is the standard approach for tumours in the lower two thirds.

Poor 5-year survival rates with surgery alone have led to investigation

Gastric cancer

- Gastric cancer is the fifth commonest cancer in men in the UK.
- *Helicobacter pylori* is a WHO-recognised carcinogen.
- Surgical resection is the only potentially curative option.
- 5-year survival rates for stage III disease are around 10%.
- A multidisciplinary approach is essential in management.

Oesophageal cancer

Oesophageal cancer is the ninth most common cancer in the UK, with over 7500 cases diagnosed each year. It is the fourth most common cause of cancer death in men, and sixth most common cause in woman in the UK, with almost 7300 deaths annually. The 5-year survival rates in men and women are only 8%. There are enormous variations in the incidence rates worldwide, with up to 40-fold higher rates in China.

Aetiology

Although tobacco and alcohol are independent risk factors for the development of squamous cell cancer (SCC), the addition of alcohol multiplies the risk from tobacco smoking. Many dietary factors have been implicated as carcinogenic, while selenium or zinc supplementation may be protective. Human papilloma virus is also documented to have increased cancer risk. Other conditions associated with increased risk are outlined in Table 1. Tylosis is an autosomal dominant condition characterised by hyperkeratosis of the palms and soles with high risk for oesophageal SCC.

Most oesophageal adenocarcinoma is associated with a premalignant condition known as Barrett's metaplasia (Barrett's oesophagus; Fig. 1). Gastro-oesophageal reflux causes chronic irritation of the oesophageal mucosa resulting in the replacement of the stratified squamous epithelium that normally lines the distal oesophagus with abnormal intestinal type epithelium (Fig. 2). Anticholinergics and other drugs which relax the lower oesophageal sphincter are associated with increased risk of adenocarcinoma as they predispose to reflux. A strong relationship has been identified between obesity and adenocarcinoma. Unlike in SCC, alcohol is not associated with an increased risk of adenocarcinoma.

Aspirin and other anti-inflammatory agents appear to protect against oesophageal cancer.

Clinical presentation

The majority of patients present with progressive dysphagia (difficulty swallowing) and weight loss. Some clinical features may vary, depending on the site of the primary tumour. Tumours involving the upper third of the oesophagus may cause hoarseness due to invasion of the recurrent laryngeal nerve, while tumours involving the lower third of the oesophagus may present with heartburn and reflux type symptoms. Patients can present with anaemia.

Pathology

Although many histological subtypes exist, the two most common are adenocarcinoma and squamous cell carcinoma (SCC). Over the last 20 years not only has the incidence rate of oesophageal cancer increased, but the ratio of the two histological subtypes has also changed. The frequency of adenocarcinoma has increased significantly in Western Europe and North America, reflecting changes in social habits, nutritional deficiencies and obesity rates.

The majority of SCCs are located in the mid-portion of the oesophagus, while adenocarcinomas tend to occur in the distal third and gastro-oesophageal junction. Lymph node involvement occurs at an early stage in both histological subtypes. Sites of lymph node involvement are outlined in Box 1.

Diagnosis and staging

Initial investigations include laboratory investigations, barium swallow and endoscopy. Endoscopy with biopsy is diagnostic. Location of the oesophageal cancer is standardised by measuring the lesion's distance from the incisors during endoscopy. CT scans of the chest, abdomen and pelvis are the minimum requirements for staging the tumour. The accuracy of CT staging may be improved using invasive procedures such as endoscopic ultrasound and laparoscopy. For locoregional cancer at or above the carina (point of bifurcation of the trachea), a bronchoscopy must be considered.

Clinical staging depends on the depth of extension of the primary tumours (Fig. 3). Although newer imaging techniques have increased clinical staging accuracy, it remains suboptimal. In a subset of patients with tumour at the gastro-oesophageal junction, laparoscopic staging is warranted.

Management

A multidisciplinary evaluation is essential, including nutritional assessment. Enteral (by mouth) nutritional support is the preferred method of supplementation. Percutaneous endoscopic gastrostomy (PEG) should be avoided in patients who may be candidates for surgical

Table 1 **Risk factors for oesophageal cancer**	
Adenocarcinoma	**Squamous cell carcinoma**
Smoking	Smoking
Higher body mass index	Alcohol excess
Gastro-oesophageal reflux	Diet poor in fruit/vegetables
Diet poor in fruit/vegetables	Achalasia
	History of gastrectomy
Barrett's metaplasia	Coeliac disease
	Tylosis

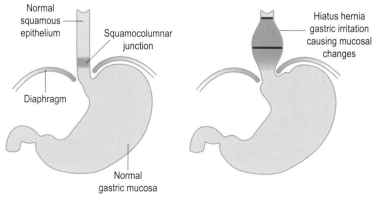

Fig. 1 **Mechanism of Barrett's metaplasia** (Barrett's oesophagus).

Box 1 *Specific regional lymph nodes*

Cervical oesophagus
- Scalene
- Internal jugular
- Upper and lower cervical
- Peri-oesophageal
- Supraclavicular

Intrathoracic oesophagus
- Upper peri-oesophageal
- Subcarinal
- Lower peri-oesophageal

Gastro-oesophageal junction
- Lower oesophageal
- Diaphragmatic
- Pericardial
- Left gastric
- Coeliac

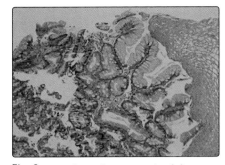

Fig. 2 **Oesophageal squamo-glandular junctional mucosa** with goblet cell formation consistent with Barrett's mucosa.

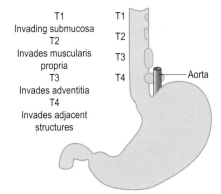

T1
Invading submucosa
T2
Invades muscularis propria
T3
Invades adventitia
T4
Invades adjacent structures

T1
T2
T3
T4
Aorta

Fig. 3 **Pictorial staging of oesophageal cancer.**

resection. A barium enema or colonoscopy should be performed if colon interposition (use of large colon in place of resected oesophagus) is planned.

Primary surgical resection has been the accepted approach but the results of surgery alone have been disappointing. Herskovic reported a landmark study using combined chemoradiotherapy showing a 25% 5-year survival with chemoradiotherapy and a 5-month improvement in median survival.

The treatment of advanced oesophageal cancer is palliative; the patient's performance status predicts whether single agent or combination therapy should be considered. Agents demonstrating some efficacy include 5-fluorouracil, platinums, taxanes, irinotecan (CPT-11) and gemcitabine.

Oesophageal stents and endoscopic laser therapy may be of some benefit to reduce symptoms of dysphagia.

Oesophageal cancer
- Oesophageal cancer is the fourth commonest cause of cancer death in men in the UK.
- Two histological subtypes exist, adenocarcinoma and squamous cell carcinoma.
- Five-year survival rates are 10% for stage III disease.
- Smoking, alcohol excess and obesity are significant risk factors for squamous cell carcinoma.
- Barrett's metaplasia (Barrett's oesophagus) is responsible for the majority of oesophageal adenocarcinomas.
- A multidisciplinary approach is essential in management.

Anal canal cancer

Introduction
Cancer of the anal canal is relatively uncommon with less than 800 cases diagnosed per year in the UK. It is more common in people who are HIV positive and in men who have sex with men, irrespective of HIV status. Its occurrence is also associated with a history of sexually transmitted diseases and smoking.

Aetiology
Human papilloma virus (HPV) has been found in over 70% of squamous cell carcinomas arising in the anal canal and is thought to play a role in carcinogenesis, as it does in cervical cancer. However, the progression from precancerous lesions to invasive cancer and the role of HPV infection has not been as clearly defined to date for anal cancer as it has in cervical cancer. In particular, the rate of progression of high-grade precancerous lesions to invasive cancer, the optimal treatment of premalignant lesions and the impact of treatment of those lesions on subsequent progression to cancer have not been elucidated.

Pathology
The anatomy of the anal canal is occasionally confused by varying uses of the terms anal verge and anal margin in the literature. These areas are illustrated in Fig. 1 and can be defined as follows:

- anal canal – the portion of the anus above the anal verge, extending upwards to the anorectal ring
- anal verge – the point at which the anal canal walls come into contact in the resting position
- anal margin – a 5 cm area of perianal skin around the anal verge.

Over 80% of anal canal cancers are squamous cell carcinomas. Previously a transitional or cloacogenic subtype was defined as originating in the transitional zone (see Fig. 1). This has now been reclassified as non-keratinising squamous cell carcinoma. Glandular elements may give rise to adenocarcinoma. Rare conditions such as melanoma and sarcoma may occur; these are not dealt with here. Squamous cell carcinomas which arise in the anal margin and do not involve the anal verge or canal should be treated as squamous cell carcinomas of the skin.

Route of spread
Anal canal cancer is predominantly a locoregional disease. Local spread may result in direct invasion of adjacent organs and denotes advanced disease. Lymph node spread occurs in 15–25% of cases at the time of presentation. The perirectal, internal iliac or inguinal nodes may be the initial sites of involvement. Distant metastases are unusual in the absence of locally advanced, uncontrolled primary disease.

History and examination
The majority of symptomatic patients present with anal bleeding. The patient may report seeing bright red blood in the toilet bowl or on the toilet tissue after a bowel motion. This may be accompanied by discomfort on sitting, pain or the sensation of a mass in the anorectal area. In advanced cases a fistula may develop between the anus/rectum and the vagina with faeces passed per vaginam. Occasionally an inguinal node may be the first symptom reported by the patient.

Digital rectal examination and proctoscopy may provide a clinical diagnosis and can be used to define the extent of the primary tumour. It may be necessary to perform the examination under anaesthesia to avoid causing pain. A careful examination for inguinal lymph nodes should be carried out. Palpable inguinal nodes harbour metastatic disease in less than 50% of cases. Therefore assessment of the nodes by fine needle aspiration and cytology is indicated prior to assigning a stage.

Pre-treatment evaluation
The acute side effects of chemoradiotherapy are potentially severe. The combination of anoproctitis and desquamation of the skin in the perineal region may make defecation very painful. Patients who have severe pain or obstructive symptoms at the time of diagnosis may benefit from a defunctioning colostomy prior to starting treatment as side effects are likely to exacerbate the symptoms.

Investigations and staging
Evaluation under anaesthesia and biopsy of the lesion will define the T stage and provide a histological diagnosis. Invasion of the vagina (T4 tumours) should be confirmed with a biopsy of any ulcerated areas seen on vaginal examination.

Routine blood tests should be done including full blood count, biochemistry and liver function tests. MRI of the pelvis is the investigation of choice in defining local extent of the primary tumour and extension to pelvic lymph nodes. The staging for anal cancer is illustrated in Table 1.

Management
The treatment of anal cancer has changed radically over the years. Historically, abdominoperineal resection was the intervention of choice. However, significant recurrence rates after surgery alone led to trials assessing the role of radiotherapy and chemotherapy. A significant proportion of patients receiving neoadjuvant chemoradiotherapy had complete resolution of their tumour prior to surgery. This prompted a move towards omitting surgery altogether for these patients. This approach has the obvious advantage to the patient of achieving cancer control without the need for a permanent colostomy.

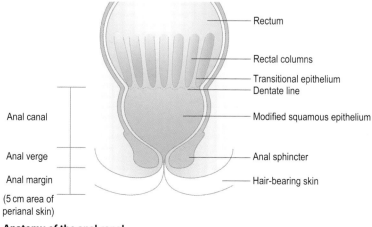

Fig. 1 **Anatomy of the anal canal.**

Rectum
Rectal columns
Transitional epithelium
Dentate line
Modified squamous epithelium
Anal sphincter
Hair-bearing skin

Anal canal
Anal verge
Anal margin
(5 cm area of perianal skin)

Table 1 Staging for carcinoma of the anal canal	
Primary tumour (T)	
TX	Primary tumour cannot be assessed
T0	No evidence of primary tumour
Tis	Carcinoma in situ
T1	Tumour 2 cm or less in greatest dimension
T2	Tumour more than 2 cm but not more than 5 cm in greatest dimension
T3	Tumour more than 5 cm in greatest dimension
T4	Tumour of any size invades adjacent organ(s), e.g. vagina, urethra, bladder. Direct invasion of the rectal wall, perirectal skin, subcutaneous tissue or the sphincter muscle(s) is not classified as T4
Regional lymph nodes (N)	
NX	Regional lymph nodes cannot be assessed
N0	No regional lymph node metastasis
N1	Metastasis in perirectal lymph nodes
N2	Metastasis in unilateral internal iliac and/or inguinal lymph nodes(s)
N3	Metastasis in perirectal and inguinal lymph nodes and/or bilateral internal iliac and/or inguinal lymph nodes
Distant metastasis (M)	
MX	Distant metastasis cannot be assessed
M0	No distant metastasis
M1	Distant metastasis

Used with the permission of the American Joint Committee on Cancer (AJCC), Chicago, Illinois. The original source for this material is the *AJCC Cancer Staging Manual*, Sixth Edition (2002) published by Springer-New York, www.springeronline.com.

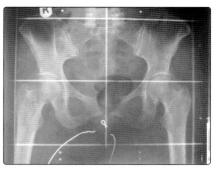

Fig. 2 **Field definitions are quite variable.** A smaller field may be used for node-negative tumours. A wide field is required to treat the inguinal lymph nodes. The wire indicates the lowest extent of the tumour.

High dose radiotherapy alone gives survival rates in excess of 70%. However, long-term side effects such as necrosis of skin within the high dose treatment area may occur. The combination of lower dose radiotherapy with chemotherapy results in similar survival rates with a more acceptable side effect profile. The side effects of chemoradiotherapy are listed in Box 1. In addition, chemoradiotherapy is associated with a higher rate of colostomy-free survival.

Chemoradiotherapy

The combination of 5-fluorouracil and mitomycin is superior to 5-fluorouracil alone and is the current standard chemotherapy regimen. The use of cisplatin in place of mitomycin is currently under investigation. A radiotherapy dose of at least 45 Gy is given concurrently by external beam radiotherapy. Fig. 2 illustrates a simulation film for radiotherapy treatment of the anal canal. A boost dose of radiotherapy may also be given. The boost may be delivered by external beam radiotherapy or a brachytherapy implant may be used.

Anal cancer is radiosensitive but responds slowly to treatment; response is usually assessed 6 weeks after completion of external beam radiotherapy.

HIV-positive patients

The toxicity of chemoradiotherapy in HIV-positive patients is poorly documented. Retrospective evidence

Box 1 *Acute and late side effects of chemoradiotherapy*

Acute side effects of chemoradiotherapy
- Bone marrow – leukopenia, thrombocytopenia
- Gastrointestinal – anoproctitis, diarrhoea, nausea
- Genitourinary – cystitis
- Skin – desquamation of the perineal skin. A severe reaction occurs in the majority of patients, often requiring a break in the chemoradiotherapy schedule to allow recovery

Late side effects of chemoradiotherapy
- Altered bowel habit with frequency and urgency
- Rectal bleeding – may occur in up to 70% of patients, 6 months after completing treatment and may last for months to years. Treatment with local steroids and/or coagulation of visualised bleeding points may help
- Ulceration and necrosis – occurs 6–18 months after completion of treatment. The incidence is closely associated with increasing radiation dose. Most cases will heal slowly with corticosteroids, antibiotics and analgesics. Surgery may be required. Differentiation from tumour recurrence is important but may be clinically difficult
- Impaired sexual function and sterility in women

suggests that toxicity is increased, particularly if the CD4 count is <200 prior to treatment. Radiotherapy and chemotherapy dose and schedules may have to be modified in this group of patients to reduce acute and late toxicity. Concomitant illness may also impair treatment tolerance. Ideally treatment should be individualised taking into consideration stage of disease, performance status and prognosis in terms of both anal cancer and HIV/AIDS.

Prognosis

The size of the primary tumour and the presence or absence of nodal involvement are significant prognostic factors. Node-negative tumours less than 2 cm in size are associated with a better prognosis.

Overall 5-year survival rates of 50–80% have been demonstrated in clinical trials. Recurrence is predominantly in the pelvis. This can be treated successfully with abdominoperineal resection and does not preclude long-term survival.

Anal canal cancer
- Carcinoma of the anal canal is relatively rare.
- It is more common in HIV-positive people and in men who have sex with men.
- Over 80% are squamous cell carcinomas.
- The majority of patients present with bleeding or localised pain.
- Chemoradiotherapy is now standard management.
- Chemoradiotherapy offers 70% overall 5-year survival.
- Recurrent disease is typically localised to the pelvis – salvage treatment with abdominoperineal resection may produce long-term survival in this scenario.

Hepatobiliary malignancies

More unusual GI tract malignancies such as hepatobiliary and pancreatic cancers are discussed in this chapter. Pancreatic endocrine cancers are discussed on page 82.

Hepatocellular carcinoma (HCC)

This is the commonest primary tumour of the liver; others include cholangiocarcinoma, angiosarcoma and hepatoblastoma. There are almost 2800 cases diagnosed annually in the UK, although it is endemic in Asia and parts of Africa. There is a male to female predominance.

Aetiology
The most common cause of hepatocellular cancer is chronic hepatitis B or C infection causing cirrhosis. The risk of HCC is also increased with other causes of cirrhosis such as alcohol, haemochromatosis and primary biliary cirrhosis. Increased relative risk is seen with toxins such as thorotrast, vinyl chloride, anabolic steroids, arsenic and aflatoxin, a mould which contaminates stored cereals.

Clinical presentation
Most patients present with late stage disease, right upper quadrant pain, anorexia, nausea, weight loss, ascites, jaundice and upper GI haemorrhage secondary to oesophageal varices. Patients may have stigmata of chronic liver disease such as palmar erythema, Dupuytren's contracture, spider naevi, gynaecomastia and splenomegaly.

Almost one third of patients will present with a solitary lesion, 60% have multiple lesions and 10% have a diffuse infiltrative process.

A rare variant of HCC, known as fibrolamellar hepatocellular carcinoma, occurs in <1% of cases. It occurs in younger, non-cirrhotic patients and is not associated with increased alpha-fetoprotein levels.

Diagnosis and staging
Serum alpha-fetoprotein (AFP) will be elevated in 30–40% of patients. Liver function tests may show elevations. Chest X-ray, abdominal CT and liver MRI are performed to assess the extent of local disease (Fig. 1).

A diagnosis of HCC is suggested with a solitary liver lesion and AFP >500 ng/dL. Preoperative biopsy is not advised with a resectable tumour for which surgery is planned as bleeding complications and seeding of the biopsy tract should be avoided. Patients are clinically staged depending on the size and number of lesions present, performance status and liver function.

Screening
Patients with risk factors for development of HCC should be screened at least annually with AFP and ultrasound. There is a lag period of approximately 18 months between abnormal findings and the development of symptoms.

Management
Only 15–30% of patients are suitable for surgery. Patients with solitary or up to three nodules <3 cm and adequate liver function should be considered for resection. Careful evaluation of cirrhotic patients is needed to determine liver reserve. The reported 5-year survival for HCC patients who undergo resection is 30%.

The role of liver transplantation is controversial, as tumour usually recurs in the graft within 6–24 months. Patients with >3 cm tumours or more than three lesions should not be considered as candidates. Palliative approaches include chemoembolisation (see Box 1 for contraindications), percutaneous ethanol ablation and radiofrequency ablation.

Gallbladder cancer

This rare cancer usually presents in the seventh decade, with a female predominance of 7 : 1. Fewer than 500 cases are seen annually in the UK. Increased risk is seen with gallstones; 80% of patients with gallbladder cancer have gallstones (Fig. 2). Risk factors are listed in Box 2.

Adenocarcinomas account for 85% of cases. One quarter present with localised disease, about one third with regional lymph node involvement and over 40% with metastatic disease. The overall 5-year survival is <5%.

Most patients have right upper quadrant pain, jaundice, anorexia, and weight loss. Ultrasound is often the first investigative modality employed and has a sensitivity of 70–100%. CT and MRI will provide accurate anatomical information and identify metastatic disease.

One fifth of patients will be diagnosed at the time of a cholecystectomy. Similar to other hepatobiliary tumours the only curative therapy is surgery. If cancer is identified at the time of laparoscopic surgery, it should be converted into an open procedure to limit risk of tumour seeding at port sites.

The role of adjuvant therapy is currently under investigation in clinical trials. Advanced disease may be treated

Box 1 Contraindications to chemoembolisation

- Hepatic artery thrombosis
- Portal vein thrombosis
- Arteriovenous shunting
- Hepatic encephalopathy
- Ascites, not controlled by diuretics
- Variceal bleeding
- Bilirubin >2.9 mg/dL
- Serum albumin <28 g/L

Box 2 Risk factors for gallbladder cancer

- Cholelithiasis
- Inflammatory bowel disease
- Gallbladder polyps
- Gallbladder calcification
- Choledochal cysts
- Obesity
- Smoking
- Nitrosamines
- Native American ethnicity

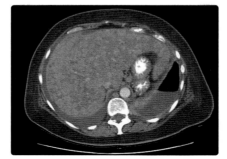

Fig. 1 **Diffuse liver involvement from HCC.**

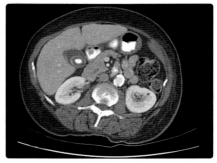

Fig. 2 **A large calcified gallstone.**

Box 3 Distribution of disease in cholangiocarcinoma

- Intrahepatic 10%
- Peri-hilar (Klatskin tumour) 40–60%
- Distal 20–30%
- Multifocal <10%

with chemotherapy; however, results are very disappointing. In the palliative setting stent placement by endoscopy or percutaneously may be of benefit.

Cholangiocarcinoma

Biliary duct carcinoma may occur anywhere along the biliary tree (Box 3). It is a rare cancer, occurring between the ages of 50 and 70 years with a slight male predominance.

Primary sclerosing cholangitis, chronic inflammation, biliary stasis, liver flukes, thorotrast, exposure to dioxin and nitrosamines are known risk factors.

It can present with right upper quadrant pain, anorexia, weight loss, pruritus, jaundice or with fevers and chills suggestive of cholangitis. Over 90% present with jaundice. Biliary duct dilatation is found on imaging studies. Medically fit, non-jaundiced patients should proceed to surgical exploration.

There is no definitive adjuvant therapy, so clinical trial enrolment should be considered in patients. Median survival for unresectable patients is 3–6 months. Although radiation and chemotherapy have been used they are of limited benefit.

Pancreatic cancer

Over 7000 new cases of pancreatic cancer are identified annually, and it is the seventh most common cause of cancer death. The median age at diagnosis is 69 years with a slight male

Box 4 Inherited disorders associated with pancreatic cancer

Familial syndromes
- Hereditary non-polyposis colorectal cancer (HNPCC)
- Breast cancer (*BRCA2*)
- Hereditary pancreatic cancer
- Ataxia telangiectasia
- Peutz–Jeghers syndrome
- Familial atypical multiple mole-melanoma syndrome (FAMM)

to female predominance. Over one third of patients have stage III/IV disease at presentation. Patients undergoing resection have 5-year survival rates of 20%, while the 5-year survival for all stages is <5%.

Aetiology
Pancreatic cancer is associated with increasing age, cigarette smoking, nitrosamines, alcohol consumption and family history. Dietary factors have been studied but no clear association confirmed. Pancreatic cancer is a disease of inherited and acquired mutations (Box 4).

Clinical presentation
Painless progressive jaundice is the most common presenting feature. Some patients have constitutional symptoms such as anorexia, back pain and weight loss.

Pathology
Pancreatic cancers may be classified as epithelial (carcinomas) or mesenchymal (sarcomas), and epithelial cancers may be further divided into solid and cystic. The most common primary malignancy of the exocrine pancreas is ductal adenocarcinoma, found in over 85% of cases. Less common variants include acinar cell carcinoma (1–2%),

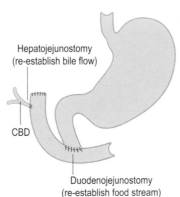

Fig. 3 **A cystic adenocarcinoma in the tail of the pancreas.**

sarcomatoid carcinoma (<1%) and undifferentiated carcinoma (<1%). Almost two thirds of ductal adenocarcinomas arise in the head of the pancreas, with only 15% arising in the pancreatic body and 5% in the tail.

Cystic pancreatic cancers may be either serous or mucinous. The mucinous variety is more common in women, presents at an early age and is associated with better survival than solid tumours.

Diagnosis and staging
The diagnosis of pancreatic cancer is based on imaging techniques and histological confirmation. CT, although useful for identifying disease location, will overestimate the potential for resection in 25–50% of cases (Fig. 3). The finding of a CA19–9 >100 units/mL in a non-icteric patient with a pancreatic mass on CT has a positive predictive value of >99%. Pancreatic cancer is staged using the AJCC TNM classification.

Management
The only curative option for pancreatic cancer is surgery; however, this is only possible in approximately 15%. The standard surgical procedure is known as a Whipple's operation (Fig. 4). This operation has a 4% postoperative mortality and complication rate of 40% in some centres. Delayed gastric emptying, pancreatic fistula and poor wound healing are examples of the complications.

Some studies demonstrate a survival benefit with adjuvant chemotherapy. Gemcitabine chemotherapy has become standard first-line therapy for metastatic pancreatic cancer.

Hepatobiliary malignancies
- Hepatobiliary malignancies are unusual cancers associated with poor prognosis.
- Surgery is the only curative option.
- Limited adjuvant therapies exist for these conditions.
- HCC with hepatitis B vaccination may be a preventable cancer in the future.

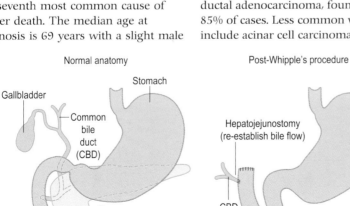

Normal anatomy

Stomach
Gallbladder
Common bile duct (CBD)
Pancreas
Duodenum

Post-Whipple's procedure

Hepatojejunostomy (re-establish bile flow)
CBD
Duodenojejunostomy (re-establish food stream)

Fig. 4 **Whipple's procedure.**

Cervical cancer

Cervical cancer is preventable. Countries which have implemented national screening programmes have seen a significant reduction in the incidence and mortality from cervical cancer. In the developing world, where access to these facilities is limited, cervical cancer is a common cause of cancer death and represents a huge burden of disease.

Aetiology

Most cases of cervical cancer are caused by infection with the human papilloma virus (HPV). HPV infection occurs in >50% of sexually active women in their lifetime – it is usually eliminated by the immune system without long-term consequences. Persistent infection with high-risk HPV (i.e. types 16 and 18) occurs in 5–10% of women. This is associated with the development of premalignant lesions which may progress to cervical cancer over a period of approximately 10 years. It is not fully understood why this happens in some women.

Risk factors for acquiring HPV infection include:

- sexual activity at a young age
- multiple sexual partners
- a high-risk sexual partner, e.g. a partner with a history of multiple partners
- history of sexually transmitted diseases.

Smoking and lower socio-economic status are also associated with an increased incidence of cervical cancer.

Pathology

Premalignant lesions are classified on the basis of increasing dysplasia into cervical intraepithelial neoplasia (CIN) 1, 2 and 3. The Bethesda system now classifies CIN 1 as low-grade squamous intraepithelial lesion (LSIL) while CIN 2 and 3 have been merged into a single category as high-grade squamous intraepithelial lesions (HSIL).

Over 80% of invasive cervical cancers are squamous cell carcinomas. Adenocarcinoma and mixed adenosquamous carcinomas also occur. Other pathological types such as lymphoma, sarcoma and small cell are rare. Cervical cancer may involve the internal and external iliac lymph nodes, the common iliac nodes, the para-aortic nodes and the supraclavicular nodes. Advanced disease may also involve inguinal nodes.

History and examination

The common presenting symptoms are listed in Box 1. Vaginal bleeding from a large cervical tumour may be torrential, necessitating resuscitation, vaginal packing and/or emergency radiotherapy to stop the bleeding.

The clinical history should describe the presenting symptoms and uncover any risk factors for HPV infection. On examination one should look for abdominal masses, hepatomegaly and inguinal or supraclavicular lymph nodes. On visual inspection of the perineum, note obvious discharge or bleeding, ulceration or abnormality of the external genitalia.

Vaginal examination should be performed with a speculum. The size and location of the tumour should be recorded. Involvement of the parametrium is determined by palpation on vaginal and rectal examination. Involvement of the vagina is determined by inspection as the speculum is withdrawn.

Investigations

- Histology – all patients should be examined under anaesthesia (EUA) to facilitate complete examination and biopsy of the tumour without discomfort. Cystoscopy and proctoscopy are also performed to identify bladder and rectal involvement.
- Laboratory tests – full blood count, renal and liver function tests may reveal anaemia due to bleeding,

Box 1 Common presenting symptoms of cervical cancer

Early stage disease
- Abnormal vaginal bleeding:
  - Postcoital
  - Intermenstrual
  - Postmenopausal
- Abnormal vaginal discharge
- Lower abdominal pain, dragging pain
- Low back pain
- Referred leg pain

Advanced disease
- Bladder involvement:
  - Urinary frequency
  - Haematuria
  - Urinary incontinence due to vesico-vaginal fistula formation
- Rectal involvement:
  - Tenesmus
  - Rectal bleeding

impaired renal function due to hydronephrosis or impaired liver function due to liver metastases in advanced disease. Women with risk factors should undergo counselling and testing to establish HIV status.
- Radiology – abdominopelvic ultrasound may identify hydronephrosis, ascites, bladder involvement, lymphadenopathy or liver metastases. The extent of the primary tumour is most accurately determined by MRI scanning, a technique that is extremely useful to ensure coverage of the tumour in planning radiotherapy treatment fields.

Staging

Cervical cancer is staged according to the FIGO staging system, which correlates with the AJCC TNM system (Table 1). This is predominantly based on clinical findings. The use of intravenous pyelogram or ultrasound to identify hydronephrosis is included; however, the use of MRI is not. Enlarged nodes or parametrial invasion identified on MRI do not alter the FIGO stage. These findings should be documented in addition to the FIGO stage.

Management

Surgery, radiotherapy and chemotherapy are all useful in the treatment of cervical cancer. The optimum modality is largely determined by the stage of disease at the time of presentation. Premalignant lesions detected as part of a cervical cancer screening programme are treated with a variety of methods.

Premalignant disease

Cervical cone biopsy refers to excision of a cone-shaped portion of cervix. Various techniques are in use, involving excision or destruction of the lesion. Treatment is routinely delivered on an outpatient basis and is well tolerated. There is no adverse effect on fertility.

Stage I

Simple surgery such as a cone biopsy (which removes the cancerous part of the cervix) or simple hysterectomy can be used for stage IA1 disease. Cone biopsy has the advantage of preserving fertility.

Stage IA2 disease carries a 5% risk of pelvic lymph node involvement and is usually treated with radical hysterectomy and lymph node

TNM categories	FIGO stages	
Primary tumour (T)		
TX		Primary tumour cannot be assessed
T0		No evidence of primary tumour
Tis	0	Carcinoma in situ
T1	I	Cervical carcinoma confined to uterus (extension to corpus should be disregarded)
T1a	IA	Invasive carcinoma diagnosed only by microscopy. Stromal invasion with a maximum depth of 5.0 mm measured from the base of the epithelium and a horizontal spread of 7.0 mm or less. Vascular space involvement, venous or lymphatic, does not affect classification
T1a1	IA1	Measured stromal invasion 3.0 mm or less in depth and 7.0 mm or less in horizontal spread
T1a2	IA2	Measured stromal invasion more than 3.0 mm and not more than 5.0 mm with a horizontal spread 7.0 mm or less
T1b	IB	Clinically visible lesion confined to the cervix or microscopic lesion greater than T1a/IA2
T1b1	IB1	Clinically visible lesion 4.0 cm or less in greatest dimension
T1b2	IB2	Clinically visible lesion more than 4.0 cm in greatest dimension
T2	II	Cervical carcinoma invades beyond uterus but not to pelvic wall or to lower third of vagina
T2a	IIA	Tumour without parametrial invasion
T2b	IIB	Tumour with parametrial invasion
T3	III	Tumour extends to pelvic wall and/or involves lower third of vagina, and/or causes hydronephrosis or non-functioning kidney
T3a	IIIA	Tumour involves lower third of vagina, no extension to pelvic side wall
T3b	IIIB	Tumour extends to pelvic wall and/or causes hydronephrosis or non-functioning kidney
T4	IVA	Tumour invades mucosa of bladder or rectum, and/or extends beyond true pelvis (bullous oedema is not sufficient to classify a tumour as T4)
Regional lymph nodes (N)		
NX		Regional lymph nodes cannot be assessed
N0		No regional lymph node metastasis
N1		Regional lymph node metastasis
Distant metastasis (M)		
MX		Distant metastasis cannot be assessed
M0		No distant metastasis
M1	IVB	Distant metastasis

Used with the permission of the American Joint Committee on Cancer (AJCC), Chicago, Illinois. The original source for this material is the *AJCC Cancer Staging Manual*, Sixth Edition (2002) published by Springer-New York, www.springeronline.com.

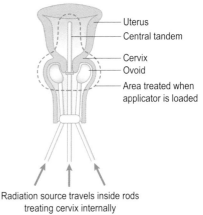

Fig. 1 **Placement of tandem and ovoids for brachytherapy treatment of cervical cancer.**

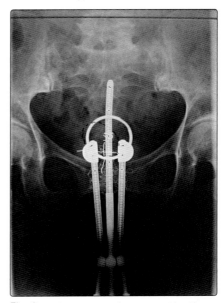

Fig. 2 **Simulation film demonstrating the position of the applicator for brachytherapy treatment of cervical cancer.**

dissection. More limited surgery such as cone biopsy and lymph node dissection may be considered if the woman wishes to preserve fertility.

Stage IB disease carries a 15% risk of pelvic lymph node involvement. It may be treated with radiotherapy or with radical hysterectomy with similar results for both treatments. Surgery involves an operative risk and may cause an atonic bladder or fistula. Radiotherapy may produce long-term side effects on the bladder and bowel and results in dry vaginal mucosa which may impact on sexual function after treatment. Unless the ovaries are removed from the radiation field, radiotherapy will induce menopause in premenopausal women. Both surgery and radiotherapy, therefore, result in loss of fertility. Some women with stage IB disease may be suitable for trachelectomy, an investigational procedure which removes the cervix, parametrium and upper vagina and can allow preservation of fertility.

Stage II and stage III

There is extensive evidence from randomised clinical trials that chemoradiation is the treatment of choice in locally advanced cervical cancer. Chemotherapy is cisplatin based and given at the same time as radiotherapy. Radical radiotherapy consists of a combination of external beam radiotherapy and brachytherapy. Brachytherapy involves the insertion of an applicator through the cervical os and placement of ovoids in the vaginal fornices. The radiation source travels through these applicators, treating the tumour from the inside. This achieves a symmetrical distribution of the radiation dose which will encompass the cervical tumour (Figs 1 and 2).

Stage IV

Palliative treatment is aimed at providing psychological and social support and relieving symptoms such as pain, offensive vaginal discharge and vaginal bleeding. Supportive measures are tailored to meet the needs of individual patients and their families.

Prognosis

Approximate 5-year survival figures are as follows: stage I disease 80–90%, stage II 45–60%, stage III 20–30% and stage IV 10–20%.

Cervical cancer

- Cervical cancer is preventable.
- Most cases of cervical cancer are caused by persistent infection with the human papilloma virus.
- Screening can significantly reduce the mortality and morbidity of cervical cancer.

- Abnormal vaginal bleeding is the commonest presenting symptom.
- Surgery is the treatment of choice for stage IA disease.
- Chemoradiation is the treatment of choice for stage II and III disease.

Uterine cancer

Endometrial carcinoma is the fifth most common cancer in women in the UK, with over 6000 new cancers diagnosed annually. It accounts for almost 5% of all female cancers. Endometrial carcinoma is responsible for 1% of cancer deaths, with over 1500 deaths annually. Its incidence increases with increasing age; median age at diagnosis is 58 years. The uterus is the site for epithelial, stromal and mixed glandular-stromal malignancies. This chapter discusses endometrial carcinoma predominantly.

Aetiology

Unopposed oestrogen exposure, endogenous or exogenous, is a common stimulus for uterine cancer development. Known risk factors are outlined in Box 1. Oestrogen exposure is suggested to be carcinogenic by causing endometrial hyperplasia, metaplasia and subsequent dysplasia.

However, a non-oestrogen-dependent phenotype exists and is characterised by a multiparous, thin woman with poorly differentiated histology and a worse prognosis. Female patients with hereditary non-polyposis colorectal cancer (HNPCC) syndrome have a 60% lifetime risk of uterine cancer.

Pregnancy reduces uterine cancer risk; there is a 30% risk reduction with the first pregnancy and 25% reduction with each subsequent pregnancy.

Smoking results in less active oestrogen metabolites, which may reduce the cancer risk.

Clinical presentation

Ninety-five per cent of patients are over 40 years at time of presentation; although 25% of patients may be perimenopausal, the most common presenting feature is irregular or postmenopausal bleeding. Therefore the majority of patients will present with early stage disease. Occasionally, atypical cells may be seen on a routine Pap smear.

Pelvic pain is a less common presenting feature. Rectal or urinary symptoms are indicative of more advanced disease.

Pathology

Endometrial hyperplasia is often a precursor lesion. The most common subtype of endometrial cancer is endometrioid. More aggressive histological types are papillary serous and clear cell carcinoma. See Table 1 for details.

Histological grading is important in determining prognosis.

Diagnosis and staging

All patients with irregular or postmenopausal bleeding should have a dilatation and curettage (D&C). Endometrial biopsy is the most reliable and accurate method of detecting endometrial carcinoma. Physical examination under anaesthesia aids in the clinical staging.

CT examination (Fig. 1) can identify anatomical information sufficient to plan surgery but MRI can provide superior images. Depth of myometrial invasion appears to be the best indicator of extrauterine spread and risk of tumour recurrence. Although TNM staging is employed, endometrial cancer can be broadly divided into localised, regional or metastatic disease (Fig. 2).

Management

Patients with endometrial hyperplasia must be followed closely with multiple biopsies, as patients may have coexistent adenocarcinoma. Even if not identified at initial testing, one third will subsequently be diagnosed with endometrial carcinoma.

Primary therapy is surgical; the surgery of choice is total abdominal hysterectomy and bilateral salpingo-oophorectomy (TAH+BSO) with sampling of peritoneal fluid for cytology.

The presence of poor prognostic factors (Box 2) highlights patients who should be considered for adjuvant therapy. Patients with stage I disease who are unfit for surgery can be effectively treated with radiation using a combination of external beam radiation and brachytherapy. All patients with stage II and III disease should be considered for adjuvant radiotherapy, to reduce the risk of local recurrence. Table 2 outlines stage-adjusted survival rates.

Patients with advanced or recurrent endometrial carcinoma should be considered for systemic therapy with either hormonal therapy or chemotherapy. Hormonal therapy in oestrogen receptor (ER)/progesterone receptor (PR) positive disease has a variable response rate between 30% and 60%. Median duration of response is less than 10 months. Chemotherapy response rates of 20% are seen with single agents.

Box 1 Risk factors for endometrial cancer

Endogenous oestrogen excess
- Older age
- Early menarche
- Late menopause
- Low parity
- Anovulatory cycles
- Obesity
- Insulin resistance/diabetes

Exogenous oestrogen exposure
- Tamoxifen
- Hormone replacement therapy
- Isoflavones – soya, grains, seeds

Others
- Hormone-secreting ovarian cancer
  granulosa cell tumour
  theca cell tumour
- Hereditary non-polyposis colorectal cancer

Table 1 Uterine cancer histology

Endometrioid adenocarcinoma	75–80%
Ciliated adenocarcinoma	
Secretory adenocarcinoma	
Papillary adenocarcinoma	
Adenocarcinoma with squamous differentiation	
Serous adenocarcinoma	<10%
Clear cell carcinoma	4%
Mucinous carcinoma	1%
Squamous carcinoma	<1%
Leiomyosarcoma	
Stromal sarcoma	
Mixed mesodermal tumours	

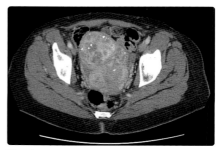

Fig. 1 **CT scan of uterine mass.**

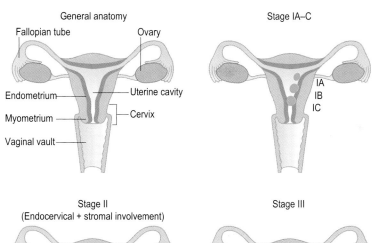

General anatomy

Fallopian tube — Ovary

Endometrium — Uterine cavity

Myometrium — Cervix

Vaginal vault —

Stage IA–C

IA
IB
IC

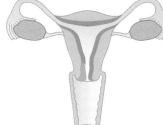

Stage II
(Endocervical + stromal involvement)

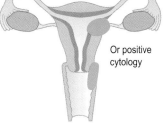

Stage III

Or positive
cytology

Fig. 2 **Staging of endometrial cancer.**

Table 2 **Stage-adjusted survival rates**

Stage	5-year survival
I	>75%
II	60%
III	30%
IV	10%

Uterine sarcoma

Uterine sarcoma constitutes 3–5% of uterine cancers. Stromal sarcomas and leiomyosarcomas arise from endometrial stroma and myometrium, while mixed mesodermal tumours (MMTs) consist of both malignant gland and stromal elements.

Uterine sarcomas present in the fifth and sixth decade.

Physical examination of patients with MMT may identify bulky tumours on bimanual examination. Distant metastases to the lungs, upper abdomen and retroperitoneal lymph nodes are common. The 5-year survival for stage I disease post TAH+BSO is <50%, with the majority of patients developing distant recurrences. However, there is no survival benefit with the addition of adjuvant radiotherapy.

Leiomyosarcoma may present with abdominal discomfort, gastrointestinal and genitourinary symptoms. Most cases are diagnosed incidentally during surgery for presumed leiomyomas. Five-year survival with stage I disease ranges from 40% to 75%. Advanced disease may show some response with anthracyclines.

Uterine cancer

■ Endometrial carcinoma is the fifth most common cancer in women in the UK.

■ The majority of patients present with irregular or postmenopausal bleeding.

■ TAH+BSO is the standard surgical approach.

■ Adjuvant radiotherapy should be considered for stage II and III disease.

■ Progestogen therapy should be considered for recurrent or advanced disease.

Ovarian cancer

Ovarian cancer represents the fourth commonest cancer among women in the UK, with approximately 7000 new cases per year. It is also the fourth leading cause of cancer death in women, with over 4500 women dying annually. The lifetime risk of developing ovarian cancer for the general population is 1.6%. Epithelial ovarian cancer (EOC) is the commonest subtype, presenting at a median age of 55–59 years. Patients with inherited ovarian cancer will present 10 years earlier and patients with non-epithelial ovarian cancer may present in the second and third decade of life.

Aetiology
Continuous, uninterrupted ovulation and menstruation causes repetitive injury to the ovarian epithelium, predisposing to genetic mutations at a cellular level and increasing the risk of carcinogenesis. Gonadotrophin excess results in epithelial proliferation, thus potentially initiating malignant transformation. Established risk factors and protective factors are listed in Table 1.

Oral contraceptive pill use for as little as 3–6 months reduces the risk of developing ovarian cancer by one third. This benefit is maintained for up to 15 years.

Up to 10% of ovarian cancers are inherited and *BRCA* mutations account for 90% of these. The presence of a *BRCA1* mutation increases the lifetime risk of epithelial ovarian cancer to 25–60%, a *BRCA2* mutation increases risk to 15–25%.

Clinical presentation
Most patients with epithelial ovarian cancer present with vague symptoms of abdominal pain and swelling. Swelling may be due to the development of extensive ascites or ovarian lesions may be 12–15 cm in diameter (Fig. 1). Indigestion, urinary frequency and weight loss also occur. Abnormal menses or postmenopausal bleeding is rare. An insidious natural history and non-specific symptoms result in the three quarters of patients presenting with advanced disease.

Germ cell tumours may present with features related to hormonal imbalances such as precocious puberty. Some patients present with an ovarian mass as an incidental finding on imaging. An ovarian mass in a premenopausal woman may be neoplastic in 6–11% of cases, while in a postmenopausal woman this risk increases to 29–35%.

Pathology
Over 70% of ovarian cancers are epithelial in nature; however, germ cell, sex cord stromal, stromal and other tumours exist. See Table 2 for the complete pathological classification of ovarian tumours. Tumours are graded as well (1), moderately (2) or poorly (3) differentiated.

A subset of epithelial ovarian cancers appears to have a better prognosis. FIGO and the WHO have designated this subset as 'borderline tumours' or 'low malignant potential' (LMP) tumours. One hypothesis suggests that these tumours represent part of a continuum of tumour progression that culminates in carcinoma. Patients presenting with disseminated 'LMP' disease may have 5-year survival rates of 70%. At present, the inability to consistently differentiate this subset can complicate management decisions.

Papillary serous adenocarcinoma is the most common EOC (Fig. 2). It is bilateral in up to 50% of cases, with psammoma bodies being pathognomonic. A psammoma body is a microscopic collection of calcium laid concentrically around a cancer cell. Clear cell carcinoma has the worst prognosis of all EOC, while embryonal carcinoma is the most aggressive of all ovarian carcinomas.

One tenth of lesions found in the ovary are metastatic deposits; the most common primary sites include gastrointestinal tract (gastric, colon or pancreas), endometrium, breast or small cell lung cancer.

Diagnosis and staging
The diagnosis of ovarian cancer requires a combination of clinical examination, imaging and surgical intervention.

- Tumour markers such as CA125 (cancer antigen 125), AFP (alpha-

Table 1 **Risk and protective factors for ovarian cancer**

Risk factors	Protective factors
Prolonged duration of ovulation	Oral contraceptive pill
Early menarche	Multiparity
Late menopause	Tubal ligation
Nulliparity	Breastfeeding
Endometriosis	
Infertility	
Smoking	
Diet – high in animal fats	
Genetic factors	
BRCA1	
BRCA2	
HNPCC (Lynch syndrome II)	

Table 2 **Ovarian cancer pathology subtypes**

Epithelial	
Papillary serous adenocarcinoma	38%
Mucinous cystadenocarcinoma	11%
Endometrioid carcinoma	13%
Clear cell carcinoma	5%
Malignant Brenner tumour	<0.5%
Undifferentiated carcinoma	15%
Sex cord stromal	
Granulosa cell tumour	2%
Sertoli–Leydig tumour	<1%
Mixed tumour	<0.5%
Germ cell tumour	
Teratoma (mature or immature)	<0.5%
Embryonal carcinoma	<0.5%
Endodermal sinus tumour	<1%
Choriocarcinoma	<0.5%
Mixed	<1%
Dysgerminoma	2%
Stromal	
Sarcomas	<0.5%
Others	
Metastatic carcinoma	10%
Lymphoma	<0.5%

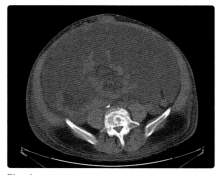

Fig. 1 **Patients may present with extensive ascites.**

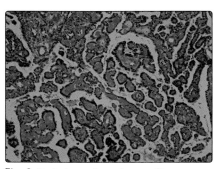

Fig. 2 **Pathology of ovarian papillary serous carcinoma.**

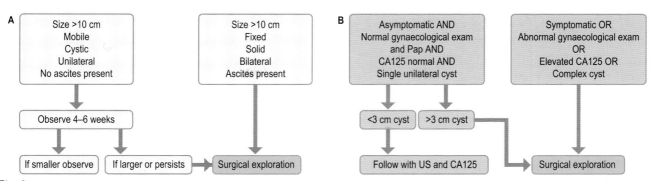

Fig. 3 **Management of ovarian masses in women.** A, Premenopausal woman. B, Postmenopausal woman.

fetoprotein), βHCG (beta human chorionic gonadotrophin) or LDH (lactate dehydrogenase) are non-specific and cannot be used as a diagnostic test. If significantly raised at diagnosis, they are useful as markers of response to treatment and relapse in the follow-up period.

- Ultrasound is a valuable tool in the evaluation of adnexal masses – documenting size, consistency and vascularity. Figs 3A and 3B illustrate the management of an ovarian mass in a pre- and a postmenopausal woman.
- Fine needle aspiration of ovarian lesions is not advised because of risk of tumour seeding.
- Surgical staging: appropriate surgical staging includes total abdominal hysterectomy, bilateral salpingo-oophorectomy, careful examination of all peritoneal surfaces, random biopsies of clinically uninvolved areas, biopsy of para-aortic nodes, cytological smear of the undersurface of both diaphragms and peritoneal washings.
- CT scans of the thorax and abdomen identify potential liver and lung metastases.

The FIGO staging (Table 3) is based on the findings at clinical examination and at surgical exploration. One quarter of patients present with early stage disease (stages I and II) and the remainder have advanced disease (stages III and IV).

Management
Optimal management depends on the age of the patient, reproductive plans, and stage of the disease. Surgery alone may be curative in stage I disease; more advanced disease requires adjuvant therapy. In stage III and IV disease, optimal cytoreduction results in a survival advantage. Optimal cytoreduction is defined as residual disease <1 cm.

Table 3	**FIGO staging for primary ovarian carcinoma**
Stage I	Limited to the ovary
Stage IA	Limited to one ovary, capsule intact, no tumour on external surface of ovary or positive peritoneal washings
Stage IB	Limited to both ovaries; capsule intact, no tumour on external surface of ovary or positive peritoneal washings
Stage IC	Stage 1A or 1B with tumour on the external surface of the ovary, ruptured capsule or positive peritoneal washings
Stage II	Limited to one or both ovaries and pelvis
Stage IIA	Extension and/or metastases to the uterus and/or tubes
Stage IIB	Extension to other pelvis tissues
Stage IIC	Either stage IIA or IIB and tumour on external surface of ovary, capsule ruptured or positive peritoneal washings
Stage III	Limited to abdominal cavity without true visceral involvement
Stage IIIA	Tumour grossly limited to true pelvis with negative nodes but with histologically confirmed microscopic seeding of abdominal peritoneal surfaces
Stage IIIB	Tumour grossly limited to true pelvis with negative nodes but with confirmed implants on abdominal peritoneal surfaces, none greater than 2 cm
Stage IIIC	Abdominal implants >2 cm and/or positive retroperitoneal or inguinal lymph nodes
Stage IV	Distant metastases such as parenchymal liver lesions. If pleural effusion is present, there must be positive cytology

Heintz APM, Odicino F, Maisonneuve P, Quinn MA, Benedet JL, Creasman WT, et al. Carcinoma of the Ovary. 26th Annual Report on the Results of Treatment in Gynecological Cancer. Int J Gynecol Obstet 2006;95(Suppl 1):S163.

The concept of adjuvant chemotherapy depends on the stage and grade of the tumour.

- There appears to be no additional benefit in patients with stage IA, grade 1 ovarian cancer.
- The addition of platinum-based chemotherapy to stage IC disease of any grade or stage II, grade 3 disease produces a 50% reduction in disease relapse.
- Chemotherapy in advanced stage disease results in superior progression-free and overall survival rates.

The current gold standard chemotherapy regimen is a combination of paclitaxel and carboplatin. The role of intraperitoneal (IP) chemotherapy has been investigated; a recent trial demonstrated that IP therapy may benefit a subset of patients with optimal debulking but results in significant toxicity.

Radiotherapy has been superseded by chemotherapy in the adjuvant setting. Its role lies in palliation of symptoms in patients whose disease no longer responds to chemotherapy.

Prognosis
The 5-year survival for ovarian cancer treated with surgery and/or chemotherapy varies widely with the stage of disease: stage I 90–95%, stage II 80%, stage III 15–30% and stage IV <5%.

Ovarian cancer
- Ovarian cancer is the fourth commonest cancer in women and the fourth leading cause of cancer death.
- 75% of patients present with advanced stage disease (stages III and IV).
- No effective screening programme exists.
- The pathognomonic feature of EOC is the psammoma body.
- Treatment is based on stage of disease, histological grade and performance status of the patient.
- Optimal surgery results in a survival advantage.
- The gold standard first-line chemotherapy combination is paclitaxel and carboplatin.

Lower tract gynaecological cancers

Lower tract gynaecological malignancies are rare; both vulval and vaginal cancers are discussed in this chapter.

Cancer of the vulva

Almost 1000 cases of vulval cancer are diagnosed each year in the UK. The 5-year survival rates are as high as 60%, as many patients present with early stage disease. Median age at presentation is 65 years, with a peak incidence around 75 years.

Aetiology

Evidence that human papilloma virus (HPV) played a role in cervical cancer led investigators to look for it in vulval cancer. Serotype 16 was found in 30–50% of cancer patients, while it was identified in 90% of patients with vulval intraepithelial neoplasia (VIN). Genital herpes virus type II and HIV are associated with increased risk. In vulval squamous cell carcinoma, two phenotypes appear to exist, depending on HPV exposure. HPV-positive tumour patients are younger, belong to lower socio-economic classes, are smokers, and the tumours are associated with VIN, are multifocal and have less keratin. In contrast, HPV-negative cancer patients are often older, the tumour is associated with vulval inflammation or lichen sclerosis, and tumours are well differentiated with abundant keratin formation.

Women who smoke and have a history of genital warts have a 35-fold increased cancer risk.

Clinical presentation

Most women present with pruritus and a palpable lesion. The lesion may be raised fleshy nodules (red, pink or white). Patients with multifocal disease can cause some diagnostic difficulties. If a lesion is neglected, women may present with local pain, bleeding or even inguinal adenopathy.

The majority of lesions involve the labia majora or minora (70%), but it may also be found to involve the clitoris (10%) or perineum (10%). Even minimally invasive cancers spread to the regional lymph nodes. The lungs are the most common site of metastases.

Pathology

A precancerous lesion known as VIN (vulval intraepithelial neoplasia) may be found at the time of cancer diagnosis in 60% of cases. In general, VIN presents at an earlier age than vulval cancer.

While over 90% of patients are diagnosed with squamous cell carcinoma, other pathologies have been reported such as melanoma (4%), sarcoma (2%), adenocarcinoma, and verrucous carcinoma.

Diagnosis and staging

A detailed physical examination including a bimanual gynaecological examination may identify the extent of the disease; however, imaging with CT, proctoscopy and cystoscopy may also be of benefit based on clinical suspicion of disease status. Vulval carcinoma may spread by direct extension, lymphatic embolisation to inguinal, femoral and pelvic nodes or by haematogenous spread to distant areas. Fig. 1 outlines the lymphatic

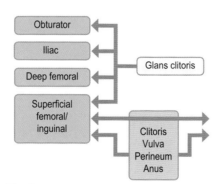

Fig. 1 **Lymphatic drainage of the vulva.**

drainage of the vulva. Surgical staging is based on the TNM classification, with size greater or less than 2 cm of importance (Table 1).

Management

Survival is dependent on nodal status; 30% of patients with operable disease have nodal disease. The primary management is surgical; however, adopting a conservative approach aiming to reduce operative morbidity and lessen body image problems is warranted. Treatment is individualised depending on the lesion size, location, depth of invasion and lymph node status. Stage 0 disease should be treated with either local excision or laser beam therapy.

Wide local excision is appropriate for stage I disease, with consideration for unilateral lymph node dissection. An alternative for those unfit for surgery is external beam radiation. All lesions of greater size require a radical complete or hemi-vulvectomy and bilateral inguinal-femoral lymph node dissections. Bilateral node dissection would not be appropriate in the management of ulcerating or fixed nodes.

In patients with more than two affected nodes, the addition of nodal and pelvic radiation improves survival. Stage III and IV disease is treated with a combination of surgery and external beam radiation. The feasibility of neoadjuvant combination chemoradiation is currently under investigation in clinical trials.

Table 1	**Staging of cancer of the vulva**	
Stage	**TNM**	
0	Tis	Carcinoma in situ
IA	T1aN0M0	Confined to the vulva or perineum, ≤2 cm in greatest dimension, negative nodes, stromal invasion no greater than 1.0 mm
IB	T1bN0M0	Confined to the vulva or perineum, ≤2 cm in greatest dimension, negative nodes, stromal invasion greater than 1.0 mm
II	T2N0M0	Confined to the vulva or perineum, ≥2 cm in greatest dimension, negative nodes
III	T3N0M0 T3N1M0 T1N1M0 T2N1M0	Tumour of any size with adjacent spread to the lower urethra or anus and/or unilateral regional lymph node metastasis
IVA	T1–4N2M0	Tumour invades any of the following: upper urethra, bladder or rectal mucosa, pelvic bone or bilateral regional nodes metastasis
IVB	Any T, any N, M1	Any distant metastasis including pelvic lymph nodes

Used with the permission of the American Joint Committee on Cancer (AJCC), Chicago, Illinois. The original source for this material is the *AJCC Cancer Staging Manual*, Sixth edition (2002) published by Springer-New York. www.springeronline.com.

Vaginal cancer

There are only about 200 cases of vaginal cancer in the UK per year, representing less than 1% of all cancers affecting women. Median age at diagnosis is 60 years. These patients often present at an early stage and therefore have excellent 5-year survival.

Aetiology

The risk factors for vaginal cancer are outlined in Box 1.

Diethylstilbestrol (DES) administered to prevent miscarriage in pregnant women until the 1970s has been associated with clear cell adenocarcinoma. It occurs in daughters of DES users, usually with onset in the second or third decade. Around 1 in 1000 women taking DES went on to develop clear cell adenocarcinoma.

Clinical presentation

Abnormal vaginal bleeding is the presenting symptoms in 50–75% of cases. More advanced disease may present with discharge and pelvic pain. Vaginal cancers occur more commonly on the posterior wall of the upper third of the vagina. Due to the complicated vaginal lymphatic drainage, a variety of different nodal stations may be involved depending on location of the primary disease.

Pathology

Different cancers may be identified in the vaginal vault; secondary involvement from cervix; vulva, endometrium and colon are not uncommon. Most primary vaginal cancers are squamous cell (85%) in origin. Adenocarcinoma (15%) has a peak incidence in the late teens. Rarely, melanoma and sarcoma are

---

Box 1 Risk factors for vaginal cancer

- HPV infection
- Genital herpes type 2 virus
- HIV
- Vaginal intraepithelial neoplasia
- CIN or cervical cancer
- Chronic vaginitis
- Diethylstilbestrol (DES)
- Pelvic radiation
- Smoking

---

described as primary vaginal cancers. Adenosquamous carcinoma is a rare and aggressive mixed epithelial tumour comprising approximately 1% to 2% of cases.

Diagnosis and staging

Speculum examination and palpation of the vaginal vault are essential components of the diagnostic work-up, as is bimanual pelvic and rectal examination. Chest X-ray, CT scan and possibly pelvic MRI are baseline investigations.

Staging is performed with the patient under general anaesthesia. The most significant factor influencing prognosis is clinical stage, reflecting depth of penetration into the vaginal wall and surrounding tissues. Scattered reports suggest superior prognosis with upper vaginal vault tumours.

Box 2 Poor prognostic factors with vaginal cancer

- Disease stage
- Age >60 years
- Symptomatic at diagnosis
- Middle or lower third vaginal vault lesions
- Poorly differentiated tumours
- Vaginal wall length involvement

Management

Treatment plans should be individualised depending upon the location, size and clinical stage of the tumour. However, radiation is the approach for most vaginal cancers. Surgery is reserved for treatment of radiation failures or lesions of the upper vaginal fornices for which radical hysterectomy and pelvic lymphadenectomy could be considered. Early stage disease can be treated with brachytherapy, while more advanced disease requires both external beam radiation and brachytherapy. Certain factors are associated with a poor prognosis (Box 2).

Chemotherapy has not been shown to be curative, thus there are no standard drug regimens. Most recurrences are in the first 2 years following treatment. In centrally recurrent vaginal cancers, some patients may be candidates for pelvic exenteration or irradiation.

Lower tract gynaecological malignancies

- Carcinoma of the vulva is associated with a history of genital warts.
- Most patients have a history of prolonged vulval irritation.
- Management of early vulval cancers is surgery.
- Radiation is the approach for most vaginal cancers.

Gestational trophoblastic disease

Gestational trophoblastic disease (GTD) is a heterogeneous group of diseases derived from an aberrant fertilisation event. There are four distinct types – hydatidiform mole (complete or partial), a benign process, and the neoplastic trophoblastic disorders: persistent/invasive gestational trophoblastic disease, choriocarcinoma and placental site trophoblastic tumours.

Hydatidiform mole (molar pregnancy)

In the UK 1 in 1000 pregnant women develop molar pregnancies, while the incidence is three-fold higher for Asian women.

Aetiology

There is a bimodal age distribution with peaks at early (<20 years) and late (>40 years) gestational age. A history of one molar pregnancy increases the risk of a second 20–40-fold, while prior miscarriage risk increases the risk three- to four-fold. Other risk factors for GTD are outlined in Box 1.

Pathology

Molar pregnancies are divided into partial or complete by different morphologic, cytogenetic and clinicopathological characteristics (Table 1).

Clinical presentation

These patients present with vaginal bleeding during the first 16 weeks, large-for-dates uterine size, hyperemesis (<10%), or passing of 'grape like vesicles' per vagina. Biochemical hyperthyroidism may be found in over one quarter of patients; as both beta human chorionic gonadotrophin (βHCG) and thyroid-stimulating hormone share an alpha subunit, the elevated βHCG may lead to rises in thyroxine.

Diagnosis

These women will have βHCG levels far exceeding those of normal pregnancy (Fig. 1). Ultrasound may simply show an enlarged-for-dates uterus or the classic 'snowstorm appearance' and absent fetus.

Laboratory investigations at baseline should include CBC, coagulation profile, blood typing, thyroid function tests, urinalysis, serum βHCG and chest X-ray.

Management

In those wishing to maintain fertility, suction evacuation with gentle curettage may be sufficient in 80–85% of patients. For patients who have completed childbearing, hysterectomy will be effective in 95% of cases. In spite of surgical therapy, a proportion of patients proceed to develop post-molar trophoblastic disease. It is imperative to monitor patients closely.

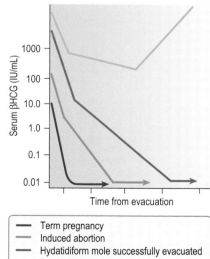

Fig. 1 **βHCG trends.**

- — Term pregnancy
- — Induced abortion
- — Hydatidiform mole successfully evacuated
- — Persistent trophoblastic disease

Serum βHCG values should be monitored weekly until there have been three consecutive normal values, and thereafter monthly for 6 months. Most patients will normalise βHCG values after 8 to 12 weeks.

Gestational trophoblastic neoplasia

This group of conditions consists of the invasive mole, choriocarcinoma and placental site trophoblastic neoplasia. The overall cure rate of this group of disorders is >90%; however, a delay in diagnosis or initiation of treatment can result in significant morbidity and mortality. The risk factors and modes of presentation are similar to those for molar pregnancy.

Invasive moles constitute 70–90% of this group of diseases; deep invasion of the myometrium and extension into venous channels can result in distant metastases in 15% of cases.

Choriocarcinoma represents 10–30% of gestational trophoblastic neoplasia. Half of these cases occur after a molar pregnancy, while the others occur after normal pregnancy (25%), abortion or ectopic pregnancies (25%). Similar to the invasive mole, common methods of spread are via direct extension or venous channels. The final subtype, placental site trophoblastic neoplasia, is extremely rare.

Diagnosis and staging

In the majority of cases GTD will be diagnosed after evacuation of a molar pregnancy, with βHCG plateau or rises. Rarely the diagnosis may be an incidental finding at the time of curettage or hysterectomy for abnormal vaginal bleeding. Due to its invasive nature women may present with metastatic disease: haemoptysis,

Box 1 Risk factors for GTD

- Infertility or nulliparity
- Smoking
- Blood type AB or B
- Oral contraceptive pill use
- Hypervitaminosis A
- Prior molar pregnancy

Table 1 **Characteristics of molar pregnancies**

Characteristic	Partial	Complete
Karyotype	Triploid type 69 XXY (80–95%)	Duplication of single haploid sperm 46 XX (95%) 46 XY (5%)
Villi appearance	Less dramatic involvement	Oedematous and avascular
Trophoblast proliferation	Less prominent	Present
Fetal development	May be present	Absent
Risk of neoplastic transformation	5–10%	15–20%

Table 2 Prognostic scoring index

Prognostic factor	0	1	2	4
Age	<40	≥40		
Antecedent pregnancy	Molar	Abortion	Term	
Interval months from index pregnancy	<4	4–7	7–12	>12
Pre-treatment βHCG (IU/mL)	10^3	$\geq10^3 <10^4$	$10^4 <10^5$	$\geq10^5$
Largest tumour size, including uterus	<3 cm	3– <5 cm	≥5 cm	
Site of metastases	Lung	Spleen, kidney	Gastrointestinal tract	Brain, liver
Number of metastases		1–4	5–8	>8
Previous failed chemotherapy			Single drug	≥2 drugs

Low risk is score of 7 or less. High risk is a score of 8 or greater.

With permission of: Ngan H, Odicino F, Maisonneuve P, Creasman WT, Beller U, Quinn MA, et al. Gestational trophoblastic neoplasia. 26th Annual Report on the Results of Treatment in Gynecological Cancer. Int J Gynecol Obstet 2006;95(Suppl 1):S193.

Table 4 Staging of GTD

Stage	T	M	Prognostic factor
Stage I	T1	M0	Unknown
IA	T1	M0	Low risk
IB	T1	M0	High risk
Stage II	T2	M0	Unknown
IIA	T2	M0	Low risk
IIB	T2	M0	High risk
Stage III	Any T	M1a	Unknown
IIIA	Any T	M1a	Low risk
IIIB	Any T	M1a	High risk
Stage IV	Any T	M1b	Unknown
IVA	Any T	M1b	Low risk
IVB	Any T	M1b	High risk

Table 3 TNM classification

Primary tumour

TX	Cannot be assessed
T0	No evidence of primary tumour
T1	Confined to uterus
T2	Extending to other genital structures by direct extension or metastasis

Distant metastasis

MX	Cannot be assessed
M0	No distant metastases
M1	Distant metastases
M1a	Lung metastases
M1b	All other metastases

Used with the permission of the American Joint Committee on Cancer (AJCC), Chicago, Illinois. The original source for this material is the *AJCC Cancer Staging Manual*, Sixth edition (2002) published by Springer-New York. www.springeronline.com.

pleuritic chest pain, gastrointestinal bleeding or even seizures and neurological deficits.

Any women presenting with atypical symptoms should have a serum βHCG level and if elevated a pelvic ultrasound to exclude pregnancy. Chest X-ray and CT scan of the abdomen/pelvis are recommended. For patients with neurological signs or symptoms, MRI of the brain is superior to CT.

Several classification systems are used, but the addition of a scoring system based on non-anatomical features has been found of benefit to identify high-risk patients requiring more intensive drug regimens (Table 2). As nodal involvement in GTD is very rare, there is no 'N' designation in the TNM staging; nodal metastases should be classified as M1 disease (Tables 3 and 4).

Management

Patients with early stage and low-risk disease may be treated with single agent chemotherapy, using methotrexate or actinomycin D. If the βHCG fails to decrease significantly after two cycles of therapy, alternative agents should be used. Once the βHCG normalises, two additional cycles are given to consolidate the therapy. Low-risk stage I/II disease cure rate is almost 90%. The remaining patients are usually cured with multi-agent therapy.

Patients with high-risk disease should be treated with combination therapy from the outset; the most common regimen is EMA-CO (etoposide, methotrexate, dactinomycin, cyclophosphamide and vincristine (Oncovin)).

Whole brain radiation should be considered for CNS involvement after administration of chemotherapy. Generally surgery is not considered for these highly vascular tumours, but in the face of persistent disease or uncontrolled haemorrhage it may be used.

Patients should have βHCG levels checked every 1–2 weeks for 3 months, then monthly for a year and then annually thereafter.

Gestational trophoblastic disease

- GTD disease occurs in 1 in 1000 pregnant women in the UK.
- Although a molar pregnancy is a benign disease, it increases the subsequent risk of neoplastic GTD.
- Careful follow-up and early therapy ensure cure.
- Non-anatomical prognostic factors are highly important in dictating therapy.

Kidney cancer

Kidney cancer represents 2% of all cancers, with over 6600 cases diagnosed each year in the UK. It is the tenth commonest cancer in men and the fifteenth commonest cancer in women, with a male to female ratio of 5 : 3. The median age at diagnosis is 65 years. There are 3600 kidney cancer deaths annually.

Rarely kidney cancer may arise in children; the most common type is a Wilms' tumour. There is a marked geographic variation, with a high rate in Eastern Europe compared to Asia and Africa.

Kidney cancer consists of mainly renal parenchymal tumours, known as renal cell cancer (RCC), and less frequently renal pelvis tumours such as transitional cell cancer (8%), oncocytomas, collecting duct tumours, renal sarcomas or secondary deposits.

Renal cell cancer (RCC)

Aetiology

The risk of RCC increases with age. High body mass index ratios are also associated with an increased incidence. Cigarette smoking results in a two-fold increase in cancer risk. Polycystic kidney disease, chronic renal disease and long-term dialysis are all associated with increased risk.

One per cent of renal cancers are familial; known associations include:

- Von Hippel–Lindau syndrome
- Autosomal dominant polycystic kidney disease
- Tuberous sclerosis
- Families with abnormalities on the short arm of chromosome 3 and on the p53 gene on chromosome 17.

The most common syndrome associated with RCC is Von Hippel–Lindau. It is an autosomal dominant condition characterised by bilateral and multicentric retinal angiomas, central nervous system (CNS) haemangioblastomas, renal cell carcinomas, phaeochromocytomas, islet cell tumours of the pancreas, endolymphatic sac tumours, and renal, pancreatic and epididymal cysts. Mutations in the VHL gene cause the syndrome due to abnormal or absent production of the VHL protein which is responsible for normal cell cycle progression.

Clinical presentation

Historically, the classic triad of haematuria, abdominal pain and a palpable mass were the presenting features; now this only occurs in <10% of patients. Over one third of patients present with early disease due to incidental findings on ultrasound or CT scans performed for other diagnostic purposes (Fig. 1); 25–30% of patients may present with metastatic disease.

Presenting symptoms include:

- constitutional symptoms such as fever, night sweats, anorexia, weight loss and fatigue
- painless haematuria (40%)
- paraneoplastic disorders (40%) – causing hypercalcaemia, polycythaemia, hypertension, masculinisation or feminisation
- male patients with left-sided renal masses may present with a scrotal varicocele
- right-sided renal tumours involving the inferior vena cava present with lower extremity oedema, ascites or embolic disease
- Stauffer's syndrome is a rare combination of hepatic dysfunction in the absence of liver metastases.

Pathology

The predominant cancer is adenocarcinoma with five different histological subtypes; the subtypes and cell of origin are outlined in Table 1. Clear cell carcinoma, also known as hypernephroma or Grawitz tumour, represent the majority of cases. Half of these cases show somatic mutations of the VHL gene and in a further 20%

the VHL gene is inactivated by hypermethylation.

Papillary RCC is associated with characteristic genetic changes such as trisomies of chromosome 3q, 7, 12, 16, 17 and 20 and loss of the Y chromosome. A diagnosis is established if these features are present even in the absence of prominent papillae.

Unclassified subtype is for those that do not fulfil the criteria for the other subgroups. Tumours are graded 1–4 depending on cellular differentiation; grading appears to have more significance for clear cell and papillary cell subtypes.

Diagnosis and staging

Renal masses are investigated with ultrasound or CT; ultrasound can differentiate between simple benign cysts, more complex cysts or solid masses (Fig. 2). MRI can evaluate the extent of collecting system or vascular involvement.

Surgical resection is warranted for any solid renal mass, with either a partial or complete nephrectomy, as it provides both diagnosis and definitive therapy. Excision of a mass is preferred rather than biopsy, to lessen risk of bleeding and tumour seeding.

Table 1 **Histological RCC subtype**		
RCC subtypes	**Cell of origin**	
Clear cell	Proximal tubule	70%
Papillary	Proximal tubule	15%
Chromophobe	Cortical collecting duct	5%
Collecting duct	Medullar collecting duct	<1%
Unspecified	Cortical collecting duct	

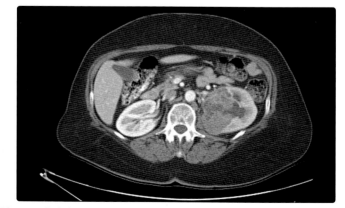

Fig. 1 **CT image of a left renal mass** upon excision pathology was consistent with a renal cell carcinoma.

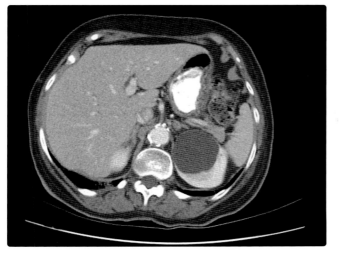

Fig. 2 **Cystic left renal lesion;** follow-up ultrasound can differentiate between simple cysts and more complex cysts.

Table 2 Staging of kidney cancer – TNM classification

Primary tumour			
TX	Cannot be assessed		
T0	No evidence of primary tumour		
T1	Less than 7 cm and limited to the kidney		
T1a	Less than 4 cm		
T1b	Greater than 4 cm but less than 7 cm		
T2	More than 7 cm but limited to the kidney		
T3	Extends into major veins, invades the adrenal gland or perinephric tissues, but not beyond Gerota's fascia		
T3a	Invades the adrenal gland or perinephric tissues but not beyond Gerota's fascia		
T3b	Extends into the renal vein or its segmental (muscle-containing) branches, or vena cava below the diaphragm		
T3c	Extends into the vena cava above the diaphragm or the wall of the IVC		
T4	Beyond Gerota's fascia		
Nodes			
NX	Cannot be assessed		
N0	No nodes involved		
N1	A single regional lymph node involved		
N2	More than one regional lymph node		
Distant metastases			
MX	Cannot be assessed		
M0	No metastases		
M1	Distant metastases		
Stage			
Stage I	T1	N0	M0
Stage II	T2	N0	M0
Stage III	T1–3	N0–1	M0
Stage IV	T4	N0–2	M0–1

Used with the permission of the American Joint Committee on Cancer (AJCC), Chicago, Illinois. The original source for this material is the *AJCC Cancer Staging Manual*, Sixth edition (2002) published by Springer-New York. www.springeronline.com.

Staging is in accordance with the TNM classification (Table 2).

Management

Prognosis depends on staging, pathological features and clinical findings (Table 3). Patients with stage I disease have 5-year survival rates of over 90%; these rates decline significantly with higher stage disease. Less than half the patients present with metastatic disease and these patients have a median survival of 18 months.

Table 3 Survival according to stage

Stage	5-year survival
I	95%
II	75–85%
III	60–70%
IV	15–25%

There are certain factors that may influence prognosis:

- Patient factors
  - symptomatic
  - weight loss >10%
  - performance status (WHO) 2–3
  - ESR >30
  - anaemia <10 g/dL
  - hypercalcaemia
  - elevated alkaline phosphatase.
- Tumour factors
  - tumour size
  - positive margins
  - multiple metastases such as liver and lung
  - high stage or grade tumour
  - sarcomatoid type
  - histological subtype.

Initial management of resectable stage I, II or III disease depends on whether renal sparing surgery is possible. Surgery may consist of either partial or complete nephrectomy. Spontaneous remission or regression of metastases is documented following surgical resection of the primary tumour but this is a rare occurrence. Surgical resection of single metastases can be curative in certain patients.

A number of adjuvant therapies have been investigated but few have demonstrated a significant survival benefit. Kidney cancer is relatively radiotherapy and chemotherapy resistant. Medroxy progesterone is a widely used hormonal agent but has minimal activity. Immunotherapy became popular due to the lack of efficacy noted with traditional therapies; response rates of 15% in metastatic RCC are seen with single agent interferon or high dose IL-2. Combination IFN and IL-2 may have response rates as high as 30–40%. In the era of new drug development with targeted therapy, VEGF (vascular endothelial growth factor) receptor inhibitors have shown activity in RCC.

Non-clear cell pathology RCC may be somewhat responsive to chemotherapy agents such as platinum, taxanes, gemcitabine or anthracyclines.

Kidney cancer

- Over 6000 new cases of kidney cancer are diagnosed each year.
- There is a male predominance.
- Increased risk of kidney cancer is associated with certain diets, smoking, chronic renal disease and familial syndromes.
- Surgery is the only curative option.
- As this cancer is relatively chemotherapy and radiation insensitive, immunotherapy and targeted therapy are proving possible therapeutic options.

Prostate cancer

Prostate cancer is the most commonly diagnosed cancer in men in the UK with an incidence of 90/100 000 per year. It is the second commonest cause of cancer death in men, being exceeded only by lung cancer. It is predominantly a disease of elderly men, and is rare in those <45 years of age.

Pathology
Most prostate cancers are adenocarcinomas derived from the glandular tissue of the prostate gland. Rare pathological types include transitional cell, squamous cell, small cell, lymphoma and sarcoma. The majority of cancers arise in the peripheral zone of the gland and can be palpated on rectal examination.

Gleason score
The Gleason score is the standard method of grading the pathological appearance of the cancer. Primary and secondary histological patterns are graded out of 5, producing a possible range of scores from 2 to 10. A Gleason score ≥8 indicates a poorly differentiated aggressive cancer.

Route of spread
Prostate cancer may spread via the lymphatics, most commonly to involve the external, internal and common iliac nodes. Distant metastases classically involve the bones but visceral metastases in the liver, brain and lungs may occur. Bone metastases preferentially occur in the lumbosacral spine and pelvis, spreading via the prostatic venous plexus.

History and examination
Early stage disease is often asymptomatic and is increasingly diagnosed by opportunistic PSA testing. Prostatism refers to a combination of symptoms caused by enlargement of the prostate gland and obstruction of urinary flow through the prostatic urethra. These symptoms include frequency and nocturia, poor stream, hesitancy and terminal dribbling (i.e. at the end of micturition).

Metastatic disease may present with various symptoms including pain related to bone metastases, a neurological deficit due to spinal cord compression or systemic upset due to hypercalcaemia.

Digital rectal examination is mandatory – it can make the diagnosis and allows clinical staging of the primary tumour. Malignant enlargement of the prostate is hard, nodular and asymmetrical and may demonstrate extracapsular extension or invasion of the seminal vesicles or rectal wall. Benign enlargement by contrast is classically smooth and softer with no extraprostatic extension.

Investigation and staging

PSA testing
PSA is a glycoprotein used as a tumour marker for prostate cancer. It is produced by both normal and malignant prostate tissue. PSA levels increase in the presence of cancer in proportion to the burden of disease. It is useful in many aspects of prostate cancer management including:

- diagnosis
- treatment decisions
- monitoring response to therapy – an elevated PSA level will return to normal 1–2 months after successful surgery and 1–2 years after successful radiotherapy treatment
- detection of recurrence or progressive disease during follow-up
- screening – although increasingly used on an opportunistic basis, evidence proving that PSA screening reduces mortality is still awaited.

Histology
Needle biopsy of the prostate gland with transrectal ultrasound guidance (TRUS) is the standard method of obtaining a biopsy sample. A sextant biopsy sampling six areas of the prostate is usually performed. This reduces the chances of missing a cancer although the false negative rate remains at approximately 10%.

Laboratory tests
Routine blood tests, bone profile and PSA should be checked.

Radiology
- CT scanning of the pelvis is commonly used to ascertain the extent of cancer within the pelvis, although MRI may provide superior staging of the primary tumour.
- Radionuclide bone scans provide images of the entire skeleton and are used to detect bone metastases. Equivocal lesions may be assessed using MRI, which is superior to bone scan in diagnosing bone metastases. Plain films may show the typical 'cotton wool' appearance of sclerotic bone lesions due to metastatic prostate cancer (Fig. 1).

Management
The potential treatment options for prostate cancer are listed in Box 1.

Early stage disease may be treated with radical nerve-sparing prostatectomy or radical radiotherapy. There are no published studies comparing these treatments directly, but the literature suggests equivalent outcome. There is a significant difference in side effect profile (Box 2).

Radiotherapy may be delivered by external beam CT-planned 3D conformal radiotherapy or by brachytherapy. External beam treatment may take up to 7 weeks to deliver the required dose. Brachytherapy involves insertion of

---

Box 1 Treatment options in prostate cancer

- Surgery – radical nerve-sparing prostatectomy
- Radiotherapy – external beam radiotherapy or brachytherapy
- Hormonal manipulation
  Surgical – orchidectomy
  Medical:
  - Gonadotrophin-releasing hormone agonists
  - Anti-androgens
  - Others
- Chemotherapy
- Watchful waiting

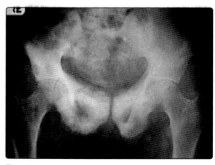

Fig. 1 **Cotton wool appearance** of sclerotic bone metastases typical of advanced prostate cancer.

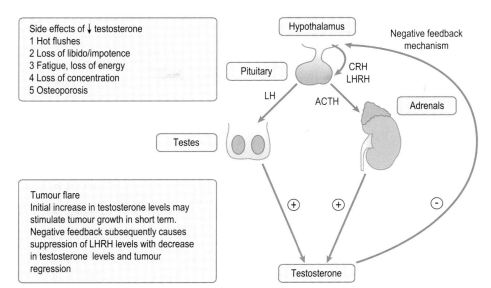

Side effects of ↓ testosterone
1 Hot flushes
2 Loss of libido/impotence
3 Fatigue, loss of energy
4 Loss of concentration
5 Osteoporosis

Tumour flare
Initial increase in testosterone levels may stimulate tumour growth in short term. Negative feedback subsequently causes suppression of LHRH levels with decrease in testosterone levels and tumour regression

Fig. 2 **Mechanism of action of the LHRH agonists.** CRH, Corticotrophin releasing hormone; LHRH, Luteinising hormone releasing hormone; LH, Luteinising hormone; ACTH, Adrenocorticotrophic hormone.

Box 2 Side effects of prostatectomy and radiotherapy

- Sexual function – higher level of erectile dysfunction and impotence after surgery
- Urinary incontinence – more common after surgery, occurring in up to 15% of cases. Occurs in 3–4% of patients after radiotherapy
- Bowel function – urgency and rectal bleeding are late side effects of radiotherapy. This does not occur after surgery

radioactive seeds within the prostate tissue. It can be performed on a day case basis, saving a significant amount of time for the patient. However, not all patients are suitable for this procedure.

Watchful waiting is a policy of non-intervention with strict monitoring. Treatment is initiated if and when disease progresses. This approach may be used in men >75 years of age with a life expectancy less than 10 years who have very low-risk prostate cancer on the basis that treatment of the prostate cancer is unlikely to prolong survival.

The optimal treatment for locally advanced tumours is under investigation. The majority of these patients are treated with radiotherapy combined with neoadjuvant or adjuvant systemic hormonal treatment.

Metastatic prostate cancer
First-line treatment with luteinising hormone releasing hormone (LHRH) agonists produces a response in the majority of patients which lasts approximately 12–18 months. The mechanism of action of these agents is illustrated in Fig. 2. Patients should be started on an anti-androgen prior to commencing LHRH therapy to prevent tumour flare (Fig. 2). Eventually the disease will progress, becoming hormone resistant. The median survival for patients with hormone-resistant prostate cancer is 12 months. Second-line hormonal therapy (anti-androgen withdrawal, glucocorticoids) and third-line hormonal therapy produce decreasing response rates with shorter duration of response.

Until recently, no treatment was proven to increase median survival for these patients. Docetaxol-containing chemotherapy regimens have now been proven to increase median survival with figures approaching 2 years.

Treatment of bone metastases and spinal cord compression is dealt with in the relevant chapters.

Prognosis
The 10-year survival for early stage organ-confined prostate cancer is in the region of 80–90%. This is in marked contrast to the survival figures for metastatic cancer outlined above.

Prostate cancer

- Prostate cancer is the most commonly diagnosed type of cancer in the UK and the second commonest cause of cancer death.
- Gleason score, PSA level and T stage can be used to predict outcome.
- Early stage disease can be treated with nerve-sparing prostatectomy or radical radiotherapy.
- Neoadjuvant or adjuvant hormones are under investigation as an adjunct to radiotherapy.
- The majority of patients with metastatic disease will respond to hormonal therapy for 12–18 months.

Testicular cancer

There are over 1900 new cases of testicular cancer annually in the UK; over 90% of these patients are cured. It represents 1% of all male cancers, and is the most common solid malignancy affecting males between 15 and 35 years.

Almost 95% of testicular cancers are germ cell tumours (GCT). This group may be further divided into seminoma and non-seminomatous germ cell tumours (NSGCT). The remaining subtypes include sex cord stromal cell tumours, gonadoblastoma, lymphomas, carcinomas and sarcomas. Lymphomas are the most common testicular neoplasm over the age of 50 years.

Germ cell tumours

GCTs originate most commonly in the gonads but may also be found in the retroperitoneum or mediastinum. These cancers may also arise in other midline areas, such as pineal gland, paranasal sinuses or sacrum.

Seminomas usually present in the fourth decade and are defined by the absence of germ cell features (pure seminoma). Human chorionic gonadotrophin (HCG) producing trophoblastic cells may be present to a small degree but do not alter the categorisation.

Other characteristics:

- testis alone disease in 70%
- retroperitoneal lymph node disease in 20%
- metastases only in 5%.

NSGCTs present in the second and third decade and may be composed of one or a variety of histological elements (Table 1). Yolk sac elements produce alpha-fetoprotein (AFP), while chorio-carcinoma elements produce HCG; these may be used as tumour markers. Characteristics include:

- greater propensity to metastasise
- approximately one third present at each stage.

Table 1 **Histological elements of NSGCT**

Tissue subtype	Source
Embryonal cell carcinoma	Embryo
Yolk sac tumour	Yolk sac
Choriocarcinoma	Placenta
Immature teratoma	Fetal tissue
Mature teratoma	Mature adult tissue

Aetiology

Undescended testes increase the risk of testicular cancer 10-fold. Approximately 10% of testicular tumours are associated with undescended testes; one quarter of these occur in the contralateral, normally descended testis. Orchidopexy before the age of 2 appears to reduce the likelihood of malignancy. Prophylactic orchidectomy is recommended for post-pubertal patients with undescended testes.

Other risk factors are:

- Positive family history – identified in 1–3%.
- Past history of testicular cancer – cumulative lifetime risk of contralateral cancer is <2%.
- Klinefelter's syndrome is associated with mediastinal extragonadal GCTs.
- Carney's complex – an autosomal dominant condition with spotty skin pigmentation, myxomas and hormone producing neoplasms including Sertoli cell tumours.
- Peutz–Jeghers syndrome.
- HIV infection – associated with an increased risk of seminoma.

Clinical presentation

The majority of patients present with unilateral testicular swelling. Testicular pain as a presenting feature may occur in 10% of cases. Back pain may occur in those with retroperitoneal lymph node involvement. One tenth of patients may present with metastatic disease, with symptoms or signs varying depending on the site of metastases. HCG secretion may cause gynaecomastia or hyperthyroidism.

Clinical examination of the testis using the thumb and first two fingers may identify a firm or hard area. Careful palpation of the abdominal cavity may reveal hepatomegaly or masses secondary to lymph node involvement.

Pathology

Germ cell tumours usually arise from intratubular germ cell neoplasia. Classic pathological features are demonstrated in Fig. 1. Tumours composed of more than one histological type are known as mixed germ cell tumours.

Diagnosis and staging

If clinical examination reveals a testicular mass, an ultrasound is

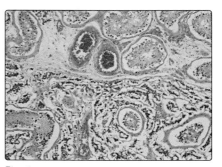

Fig. 1 **Classic seminoma (lower) with intratubular germ cell neoplasia (upper).**

warranted to distinguish between cystic and solid lesions. If a solid mass is confirmed the patient should proceed to an inguinal orchidectomy. This includes removal of the testis and ligation of the spermatic cord to the level of the internal ring, as the testis originates in the genital ridge and migrates to the scrotum. Biopsy of testicular masses should not be performed due to potential risk of seeding.

Differential diagnoses of a testicular mass include:

- testicular torsion
- epididymitis
- hydrocele
- varicocele
- hernia.

Chest X-ray (CXR) and tumour markers should be assessed preoperatively. CT scan of chest, abdomen and pelvis is standard, and imaging of brain should be considered for symptomatic or high-risk patients. Asymptomatic metastases may be identified in this manner; Fig. 2 demonstrates lung metastases on CXR and CT. Bone scan should be considered for those who are symptomatic or have elevated alkaline phosphatase.

Tumour markers

Tumour markers AFP, HCG and lactate dehydrogenase (LDH) have independent prognostic significance. The absolute value at diagnosis, rate of decline and absolute normalisation of values determine therapeutic approaches. Monitoring of serial values is essential. The half-life of AFP is 5–7 days and HCG 18–36 hours. A failure to normalise within the determined time frame is indicative of residual disease.

Staging requires incorporation of clinical findings, CT findings and

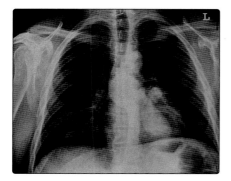

A

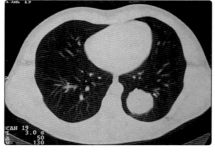

B

Fig. 2 **Metastatic lung disease.**

Fig. 3 **Residual retroperitoneal lymphadenopathy post chemotherapy.**

Table 2 **Risk classification of testicular cancer**

NSGCT	Seminoma
Good risk	**Good risk**
Testicular or retroperitoneal primary	Any primary site
No non-pulmonary metastases	No non-pulmonary metastases
Good markers: AFP <1000 ng/mL	Normal AFP
HCG <5000 units/mL	Any βHCG
LDH <1.5 × normal	Any LDH
Intermediate risk	**Intermediate risk**
Testicular or retroperitoneal primary	Any primary site
No non-pulmonary metastases	Non-pulmonary metastases
Intermediate markers: AFP 1000–10 000 ng/mL	Normal AFP
HCG 5000–50 000 units/mL	Any βHCG
LDH 1.5–10 × normal	Any LDH
High risk	No high-risk seminoma patients
Mediastinal primary	
Non-pulmonary metastases	
Markers: AFP > 10 000 ng/mL	
HCG > 50 000 units/mL	
LDH > 10 × normal	

Based upon the guidelines of the International Germ Cell Cancer Collaborative Group. JCO, vol 15(2), 1997; p 594–603.

Table 3 **Common testicular chemotherapy regimens**

Abbreviation	Drugs	Dosage	Schedule
EP	Etoposide	100 mg/m²/day	Days 1–5
	Cisplatin	20 mg/m²/day	Days 1–5
BEP or PEB	Bleomycin	30 IU/week	Days 2, 9, 16
	Etoposide	100 mg/m²/day	Days 1–5
	Cisplatin	20 mg/m²/day	Days 1–5
VIP	Etoposide (VP16)	75 mg/m²/day	Days 1–5
	Ifosfamide	1200 mg/m²/day	Days 1–5
	Cisplatin	20 mg/m²/day	Days 1–5
VelP	Vinblastine	0.11 mg/kg	Days 1–2
	Ifosfamide	1200 mg/m²/day	Days 1–5
	Cisplatin	20 mg/m²/day	Days 1–5
TIP	Paclitaxel	160 mg/m²/day	Day 1
	Ifosfamide	1200 mg/m²/day	Days 2–5
	Cisplatin	20 mg/m²/day	Days 2–5

tumour markers, stratifying patients with NSCGT into good, intermediate and poor risk categories. There is no poor risk seminoma stage (Table 2).

Management

Seminoma

Stage I disease is associated with relapse rates of approximately 10%; radiation reduces the relapse rate by half. Close surveillance or single dose carboplatin are reasonable alternatives. See Table 3 for chemotherapy regimens.

Stage II disease with adenopathy greater than 5 cm should receive adjuvant chemotherapy (BEP × 3 cycles or EP × 4 cycles); however, if the nodal mass is <5 cm adjuvant radiation alone may be sufficient. All stage III disease should receive chemotherapy (BEP 3–4 cycles). Residual masses may be observed post therapy.

NSGCT

The risk of recurrence with clinical stage I disease is 20–30%, but if it recurs >95% of patients are curable;

therefore close observation is a possible option. If close observation is not possible, retroperitoneal lymph node dissection (RPLND) could be considered and if positive nodes are found adjuvant chemotherapy is indicated.

Stage II disease with masses >3 cm should receive chemotherapy. Those with nodes <3 cm may proceed to RPLND or chemotherapy. If patients are unable to take bleomycin (asthmatics, smokers, Raynaud's phenomenon, vascular disease), VIP is indicated.

Post-chemotherapy surgery is critical in the management of patients with residual masses. See Fig. 3 for an example of persistent retroperitoneal lymph node disease post chemotherapy. For NSGCT any residual abnormality should be resected – 20–30% will be viable germ cell elements, 25–30% mature teratoma and 50% necrotic debris.

Toxicity of therapy

As this cancer is highly treatable it is very important to be aware of all the potential treatment-related toxicities. Sperm banking should be offered to all patients prior to starting therapy. This may be technically difficult as sperm counts may be low related to the disease. Risk of pulmonary toxicity with bleomycin must be considered. There is a small (<0.5%) but definite risk of chemotherapy-induced leukaemia. RPLND can be associated with operative morbidities, retrograde ejaculation and urinary tract damage.

Testicular cancer

- Represents 1% of all male cancers.
- Two main categories are seminoma and NSGCT (non-seminomatous germ cell tumours).
- Even at advanced stage disease, it remains highly curable.
- Close monitoring of tumour markers is essential post therapy.
- Awareness of long-term treatment toxicities is warranted.

Other genitourinary cancers

Genitourinary cancers not described elsewhere include bladder cancer, penile and urethral cancer.

Bladder cancer

Bladder cancer represents the fourth most common malignancy in men, with over 11 000 new cases per year in the UK, and the tenth most common cancer in women. It causes just under 5000 cancer deaths per year. The incidence of bladder cancer continues to increase but the survival figures remain stable.

Aetiology

There is a close relationship between bladder cancer risk and smoking. Carcinogens include:

- aromatic amines found in rubber, leather, paint, chemical and petroleum industry; exposure increases the risk 60-fold
- tobacco exposure – cigars, pipe smoking and second hand smoke
- *Schistosoma haematobium*
- chronic bladder infection
- Balkan nephropathy – a corona virus-mediated disease found in Balkan countries
- arsenic poisoning.

Pathology

Bladder cancer arises from the urothelium lining the renal tract. Over 90% of cases are transitional cell carcinoma (TCC) (Fig. 1); other types seen include squamous cell carcinoma (8%), adenocarcinoma (<2%) and rhabdomyosarcoma (<1%).

Histological evaluation should include a description of the cell type, grade (1–3), and depth of invasion. Multiple lesions are seen in over half the patients.

Certain molecular features have been recently identified:

- 60% have deletions of cell proliferation regulators *p15* or *p16* on chromosome 9
- abnormal expression of *p53*
- abnormal expression of the *RB* gene
- Oncogenes such as *RAS* and *cerb-B2* are activated.

Clinical presentation

Eighty per cent of patients present with painless haematuria which may be gross or microscopic. One third of patients

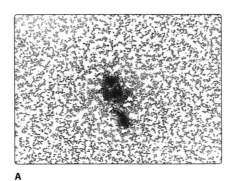
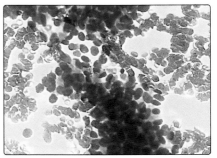

Fig. 1 **Transitional cell cancer of the bladder under low (A) and high (B) power.**

will have urinary urgency, frequency, or dysuria. Stage IV disease presentation occurs in about 5% of cases with symptoms such as weight loss, abdominal mass, flank pain or lymphoedema.

Diagnosis and staging

Cytological analysis of urine may result in the diagnosis in 50–90% of cases. Suspicious symptoms should be investigated with cystoscopy. Biopsy of all suspicious lesions and adjacent areas should be performed.

CT scan of the abdomen/pelvis, bone scan (if symptomatic or elevated alkaline phosphatase) and intravenous pyelography (IVP) are helpful in staging the disease. IVP is capable of identifying upper renal tract cancers, which occur in 2–3% of cases.

Staging is performed using the TNM classification but one of the most important factors is the degree of invasiveness. Ta lesions (not invading the lamina propria) have a subsequent risk of invasion or metastasis of 9% versus 29% for those that do invade the lamina propria (T1) (Fig. 2).

Management

Traditionally it is divided into three major categories: superficial, invasive and metastatic disease, each associated with different survival rates.

Superficial

Superficial bladder cancer occurs in 80% of patients and the mainstay approach is transurethral resection. However, recurrence is not uncommon in T1 lesions; adjuvant intravesical chemotherapy is known to reduce the recurrence risk. Thiotepa, mitomycin C, doxorubicin and epirubicin have all been used with some benefit.

Patients may also receive immunotherapy with intravesical BCG;

this weekly instillation can provide long-term protection. It must not be initiated immediately after bladder resection or if the patient has had recent traumatic urinary catheterisation as these increase the risk of systemic BCG dissemination.

Three-monthly cystoscopy is required to follow these patients and identify recurrences early.

Locally advanced

There are no randomised controlled trials to guide treatment choice in patients with locally advanced disease. The choice remains between radical radiation and radical cystectomy. Retrospective review documents 5-year overall survival rate for surgery as 40–50% while it is 35–40% for radiation.

Systemic chemotherapy has been incorporated with definitive radiation therapy to develop a more effective bladder-sparing approach for patients with locally advanced disease.

Metastatic bladder cancer can be treated with combination chemotherapy (MVAC methotrexate, vinblastine, adriamycin and cisplatin); however, this aggressive regimen is associated with significant toxicities, particularly haematological. It results in a response rate of 39% and a median survival of 12 months. Newer agents as single agents (taxanes, ifosfamide and gemcitabine) are currently under review.

Penile cancer

Only about 350 men are diagnosed with penile cancer annually in the UK. Most patients present in their seventh decade. This rare cancer has been associated with HPV infection, particularly serotypes 16, 18, 31 and 33, ultraviolet phototherapy, and

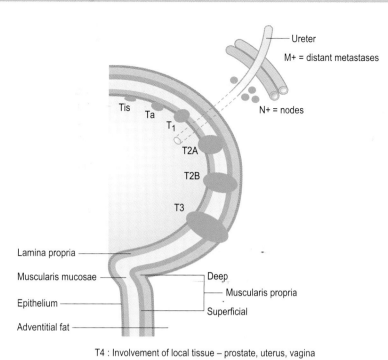

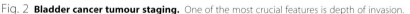

T4 : Involvement of local tissue – prostate, uterus, vagina

Fig. 2 **Bladder cancer tumour staging.** One of the most crucial features is depth of invasion.

phimosis, while circumcision has a protective effect.

Clinical presentation

A small lesion causing ulceration, irritation or bleeding is usually the presenting complaint. More than half the patients will delay seeking medical attention due to embarrassment. Metastatic disease at presentation is very rare.

Pathology

SCC occurs in 95% of cases, while the remaining cancers consist of sarcoma, basal cell carcinomas and melanoma.

Diagnosis and staging

The diagnosis is established by biopsy of any suspicious lesion. Routine staging includes chest X-ray and CT of the abdomen/pelvis. Non-invasive staging is inaccurate; at most up to one third of palpable nodes may be enlarged due to infection or inflammation. Depth of invasion is the most useful prognostic indicator of lymph node involvement. The AJCC has designated staging by the TNM classification.

Five-year survival rates vary significantly between stages:

- Stage I – 90%
- Stage II – 66%
- Stage III – 24%
- Stage IV – 5%.

Management

Carcinoma in situ of the penis may be treated with surgical excision but this can be associated with scarring, deformity and impaired function. Other therapeutic options include topical 5-fluorouracil, imiquimod 5% cream (a topical immune response modifier), laser therapy with Nd: YAG, CO_2 lasers or cryosurgery.

For lesions limited to the foreskin, wide local excision with circumcision may be adequate therapy for control. For infiltrating tumours of the glans, penile amputation or radiation should be employed. For those in whom surgery is planned, lymphadenectomy should be considered after discussion with the patient outlining the associated complications. Radiation to lymph node areas may be given to those unsuitable for surgery. No standard therapy exists for metastatic disease.

Urethral cancer

The majority present in their late 50s. Anatomical differences between the sexes result in subtle differences in the disease entity. This is the only urological malignancy occurring at greater frequency in women than men.

Clinical presentation

The onset of disease is insidious; the interval between the onset of symptoms and diagnosis may be as long as 3 years. Tumours of the penile urethra present with irritative or obstructive voiding symptoms. Anterior lesions may present a palpable mass. Lesions of the prostatic urethra may present with urinary symptoms.

In female patients bleeding is the most common complaint and a mass may be detectable on examination.

Pathology

The most common histological subtype is SCC, except in the prostatic urethra where cancers are TCC. Adenocarcinoma, melanoma, undifferentiated carcinoma occur less frequently.

Diagnosis

Diagnosis is made by urethroscopic biopsy. Baseline investigations include serum chemistries, chest X-ray, CT of the abdomen/pelvis. Fine needle aspiration of suspicious lesions is recommended. The prognosis of urethral cancer depends on its anatomical location and the depth of invasion.

In females, the most common sites of tumour invasion are the labia, vagina and bladder neck. In males, the most common sites of extension are the vascular spaces of the corpora and periurethral tissues, the deep tissues of the perineum, the urogenital diaphragm, the prostate, and the penile and scrotal skin, where it causes abscesses and fistulae.

Management

Surgery is indicated to confirm a diagnosis of clinically suspected urethral cancer. More extensive surgery is indicated for local control of a primary urethral neoplasm and is dependent on the size, location and extent of the tumour and the overall condition of the patient. Even with this approach, local recurrences are significant, so adjuvant radiation has been suggested to reduce this risk. The addition of radiation is not without toxicity: incontinence, local fistula, stricture, abscess, cystitis and cellulitis.

In general, the benefit of prophylactic lymphadenectomy is not proven and is associated with significant morbidity. Chemotherapy or combined modality approaches are currently under investigation for this rare cancer.

Other genitourinary cancers

- Bladder cancer is a common malignancy.
- Although 80% of patients are stage I at presentation, there is a high local recurrence rate and local adjuvant therapies should be employed.
- Prompt attention to haematuria is important.
- More effective therapies are needed.

Head and neck cancer – 1

The term head and neck cancer refers to a group of cancers derived from distinct primary sites within the head and neck (Box 1 and Fig. 1). Knowledge of the anatomy of the region is required to distinguish between primary sites, stage disease correctly and appreciate technical aspects of treatment procedures. Many of these cancers share aetiological factors, have overlapping presenting symptoms, and are treated with similar modalities.

Epidemiology

The risk of head and neck cancer increases with age. It is generally more common in men than in women, as men in most societies are more likely to smoke and drink alcohol, the main causative factors. Epidemiological studies in both the developed and the developing world are showing an increase in head and neck cancer incidence.

Incidence patterns show pronounced regional variation. Nasopharyngeal cancer occurs with unsurpassed frequency in Hong Kong and South-East Asia. There is an extremely high incidence of hypopharyngeal cancers in localities in France, thought to be related to Calvados, a characteristic brandy of the region. Tumours of the oral cavity are common in the developing world in part due to the practice of chewing tobacco and betel nut.

Aetiology

Tobacco and alcohol are the major causative agents in head and neck cancers. These two agents act synergistically, probably accounting for half of all head and neck cancer cases.

Genetic predisposition, dietary and viral factors also play a role. Epstein–Barr virus, human papilloma virus and human herpes virus have all been associated with various head and neck cancers. Epstein–Barr virus is closely associated with nasopharyngeal cancer, with copies of the virus found within the malignant cells, although a causative mechanism has not been elucidated.

Pathology

While the tissues within the head and neck region may give rise to tumours of diverse histology, both benign and malignant, squamous cell carcinoma is by far the most common type. Dysplasia and leukoplakia (white patches on the mucosa) have been identified as lesions which may progress to invasive squamous cell carcinoma. Certain subsites within the head and neck are associated with a particular pathological spectrum of disease. For instance, the tonsils which form part of Waldeyer's ring may give rise to non-Hodgkin's lymphoma.

Nasopharynx

The WHO has classified three types of nasopharyngeal carcinoma:

- type I: keratinising squamous cell carcinoma
- type II: differentiated non-keratinising carcinoma
- type III: undifferentiated carcinoma.

Types II and III are alike in terms of presentation and treatment. Undifferentiated carcinoma (Fig. 2) is the most common subtype occurring in areas of high incidence such as South-East Asia. It is this subtype that is associated with the Epstein–Barr virus.

Salivary gland cancers

The major salivary glands consist of paired parotid, submandibular and sublingual glands. The minor salivary glands are scattered throughout the mucosa of the mouth. The most common tumour in the salivary glands is benign – a pleomorphic adenoma. Tumours in the minor salivary glands are more likely to be malignant. Histological types are:

Box 1 Head and neck cancers – primary sites

- Lip and oral cavity
- Pharynx
  Nasopharynx
  Oropharynx
  Hypopharynx
- Larynx
- Major salivary glands
- Nasal cavity and paranasal sinuses

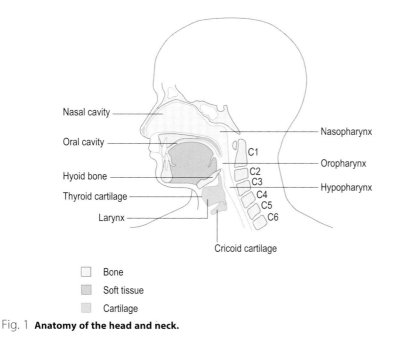

Nasal cavity
Oral cavity
Hyoid bone
Thyroid cartilage
Larynx
Nasopharynx
C1
C2
C3
C4
C5
C6
Oropharynx
Hypopharynx
Cricoid cartilage

Bone
Soft tissue
Cartilage

Fig. 1 **Anatomy of the head and neck.**

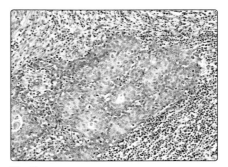

Fig. 2 **Type III (undifferentiated) nasopharyngeal carcinoma.** Courtesy of Dr David Delaney.

- mucoepidermoid carcinoma
- acinic cell carcinoma
- adenoid cystic carcinoma
- adenocarcinoma
- squamous cell carcinoma.

Typical clinical patterns of behaviour are observed with different histological types, e.g. adenoid cystic carcinoma tends to spread along the route of nerves.

Nasal cavity and paranasal sinuses

The variety of tissues within this area is reflected in the diversity of cancers which may occur. While the most common type of cancer is squamous cell carcinoma, adenocarcinoma may account for up to 20% of cases. Rarer entities include melanoma, lymphoma, sarcoma and olfactory neuroblastoma.

Second primary cancers

The theory of field cancerisation states that the entire mucosa of the upper aerodigestive tract is affected by the carcinogenic process, not just a particular location in which cancer may be diagnosed. This idea correlates well with the clinical observation that head and neck cancer patients have an increased incidence of second primary cancers, commonly occurring in the head and neck region, the oesophagus and the lung. The risk of a second primary occurring is approximately 5% per year. This event heralds a poor prognosis in spite of successful treatment of the initial primary tumour.

Anatomy

The complexity of the anatomy within the head and neck region has a profound impact on the major treatment modalities of surgery and radiotherapy. Numerous vital structures are found in a compact area vital for the performance of the basic functions of breathing, eating and speaking. Cancers which require extensive surgery or radiotherapy or both may result in significant morbidity and impairment of these basic functions. Fig. 1 illustrates the anatomical location of the major primary sites within the head and neck.

History and examination

The presenting symptoms of head and neck cancer largely depend on the location and stage of the primary cancer. Specific symptoms are dealt with in the relevant sections. Locally advanced cancer is frequently associated with difficulty eating, resulting in varying degrees of weight loss. The degree and duration of weight loss should be documented with care.

Primary tumours of the lip, oral cavity, oropharynx and nasal cavity area are easily accessible to clinical examination. Tumours of the larynx can be examined in the clinic using a flexible endoscope. No preparation is required beyond spraying anaesthetic in the nose to allow easy passage of the scope. Visualisation of the primary tumour and examination of the cervical lymph nodes will determine the clinical stage of disease.

Pre-treatment evaluation

Patients with head and neck cancer frequently have concomitant medical problems associated with smoking and alcohol consumption. Optimal management requires the active participation of a multidisciplinary team. Important issues to be considered prior to treatment include:

- Concomitant medical conditions – cardiovascular and respiratory diseases may preclude radical treatment.
- Nutrition – many patients, particularly those with advanced tumours, may be in poor general health at the time of diagnosis. Difficulty eating may have resulted in significant weight loss. An extensive surgical procedure or radical radiotherapy will compound these symptoms. Difficulties which would affect postoperative recovery or precipitate a break in radiotherapy treatment can be pre-empted by timely insertion of a PEG (percutaneous gastrostomy; see Fig. 3 on p. 61) to maintain nutrition. Early referral to an experienced dietician is mandatory.
- Dentition – teeth which are in poor condition confer a risk of osteoradionecrosis if they are within the radiotherapy treatment field. Patients should be referred to a specialist dental service prior to simulation for review and removal of teeth as necessary.

Staging

Primary tumour

All subsites are associated with an individual staging system for the primary tumour itself, based on the maximum dimensions of the tumour or its maximum anatomical extent within the surrounding tissues.

Cervical lymph nodes

The same system is used to record the size and extent of cervical lymph node involvement for all primary tumour sites except the nasopharynx. Extensive cervical lymph node involvement may be associated with a reasonably good prognosis in nasopharyngeal carcinoma unlike other subsites within the head and neck. A modified cervical node staging system is employed to recognise this fact.

Investigations

- Biopsy – definitive diagnosis requires biopsy of the primary lesion. This is a straightforward procedure when the tumour is immediately accessible. In other cases endoscopic examination under general anaesthesia allows biopsy and staging. Patients who present with an enlarged cervical lymph node may have fine needle aspiration and cytology as a first diagnostic procedure.
- Imaging – CT and MRI scans provide complementary information. While CT is superior in the diagnosis of cervical lymphadenopathy, the MRI provides improved visualisation of soft tissue involvement by the primary tumour. PET scanning is increasingly used. Distant metastases are relatively uncommon in all subsites except the nasopharynx. The most common sites of distant disease are the bones, liver and lungs.

> **Head and neck cancer – 1**
>
> - Tobacco and alcohol are responsible for the majority of head and neck cancers.
> - Field cancerisation theory states that the entire mucosa of the upper aerodigestive tract is at risk.
> - Second primary cancers occur at a rate of 5% per year in patients successfully treated for head and neck cancer.
> - Clinical behaviour of disease varies according to histological subtype and site of origin within the head and neck.

Head and neck cancer – 2

Larynx

Presenting symptoms

There are three subsites within the larynx – supraglottis, glottis and subglottis. The glottis contains the true vocal cords and accounts for the majority of laryngeal cancers. The supraglottic region is also a common site of origin; subglottic tumours being rare.

The prime symptom of laryngeal disease is a change in the timbre of the voice. Hoarseness may be mild or severe or varying in intensity over time. Glottic tumours produce hoarseness at an early stage. This combined with the fact that the true vocal cords have limited lymphatic supply means that glottic cancers are usually diagnosed at an early stage, when the disease is confined to the vocal cords and the cervical nodes are not involved.

Early supraglottic disease may cause few or no symptoms. Hoarseness does not occur with early stage disease. Dysphagia is common but mild symptoms may not be noticed by the patient for some time. This combined with a rich lymphatic supply results in frequent presentation with node-positive advanced disease (Fig. 1).

Management

Early stage disease

Both radiotherapy and voice-sparing surgery (vertical hemilaryngectomy, supraglottic laryngectomy) provide excellent overall survival in the treatment of early stage disease. In practice the vast majority of patients are treated with radical radiotherapy, which provides the best long-term

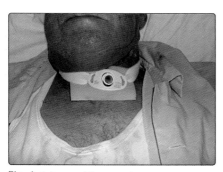

Fig. 1 **Advanced laryngeal carcinoma.** Tracheostomy in place and ulcerated lymph nodes seen on the left.

voice quality. Surgery is reserved for salvage in the event of relapse. Long-term survival with this approach is over 90% for T1 tumours and over 80% for T2 tumours.

Locally advanced disease

Locally advanced disease requires extensive combined modality treatment. A surgical approach usually necessitates laryngectomy due to the extent of the primary tumour with consequent loss of function in terms of eating and speaking.

The goal of preserving the larynx has stimulated the development of treatment protocols which allow organ preservation while maintaining similar survival rates to those achieved with laryngectomy. Wide field radiotherapy which includes the cervical lymph node areas is given in combination with neoadjuvant cisplatin and 5-fluorouracil based chemotherapy. Laryngectomy is reserved for salvage treatment in those patients who do not respond to chemoradiotherapy.

Nasopharynx

Presenting symptoms

An enlarged cervical lymph node is often the first sign of disease as the primary tumour within the nasopharynx may be completely asymptomatic. Typical symptoms such as unilateral deafness or tinnitus, nasal stuffiness or epistaxis precipitate investigation although the diagnosis of nasopharyngeal cancer may be delayed. Invasion of the skull base is frequently present at the time of diagnosis. A variety of cranial nerve palsies may occur, the most common involving nerves III to VI.

Nasopharyngeal cancer is associated with a much higher incidence of distant metastases than other head and neck cancers, the most common sites being bone, lung and liver. Full staging requires imaging of these sites prior to treatment.

Management

The high incidence of nasopharyngeal cancer in South-East Asia has led to the development of significant expertise in early diagnosis and treatment of the disease. The Ho

staging system, which differs from the TNM system, is used. Results may not be directly transferable to Western populations, however, where type I keratinising squamous cell carcinoma is the predominant type of disease as compared with types II and III in South-East Asia.

Chemoradiotherapy

There is extensive evidence showing superior results for chemoradiotherapy compared to radiotherapy alone in the treatment of locally advanced nasopharyngeal carcinoma. Cisplatin-based chemotherapy regimens have been used on a neoadjuvant, concomitant and adjuvant basis. Many patients fail to complete adjuvant chemotherapy due to the toxicity following concomitant treatment, leading some physicians to advocate neoadjuvant chemotherapy followed by concomitant treatment.

The propensity for occult nodal disease mandates large radiation fields to treat the cervical nodes on both sides of the neck as well as the primary tumour itself. Doses in the range of 60 to 70 Gy are commonly used. A boost dose to the primary tumour site may be given using brachytherapy techniques. Acute and late side effects of treatment are significant. Late side effects of radiotherapy are discussed in Head and neck cancer – 3.

Residual or recurrent disease is often treated with re-irradiation. Techniques used include external beam radiotherapy, brachytherapy and stereotactic radiosurgery. Stereotactic treatment entails precise three-dimensional planning to focus narrow radiation beams on a target area which should be <3 cm in size.

Prognosis

Survival following treatment for nasopharyngeal cancer has improved over the last three decades. Type III disease has a better prognosis, with 5-year survival rates in the region of 70%, in comparison with 40% for type I disease.

Oropharynx

The location of cancers within the oropharynx influences their

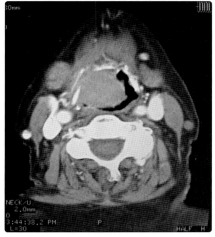

Fig. 2 **Large tumour arising in the oropharynx** extending into the oral cavity, associated with enlarged lymph nodes.

management. An early cancer in the posterior third of the tongue is usually treated with radiotherapy because surgery, although curative, will result in disproportionate loss of function. Early tonsillar lesions by comparison are easily treated with surgery. More advanced lesions (Fig. 2) are treated with a combination of surgery and radiotherapy.

Surgical procedures may be extensive, requiring a combination of glossectomy and laryngectomy for instance. External beam radiotherapy is most commonly used although brachytherapy may be used to give a boost dose to the tonsil or posterior third of the tongue. Chemotherapy may be given concurrently to improve local control.

Hypopharynx

These tumours are relatively uncommon in the UK. Hypopharyngeal tumours are usually diagnosed at a locally advanced stage because early disease tends to be asymptomatic. The proximity of the hypopharynx to the larynx means that laryngectomy is often required if surgery is considered. The organ preservation approach described above for laryngeal cancer is also used in the treatment of hypopharyngeal cancer.

Rehabilitation after laryngectomy

Treatment for head and neck cancer may produce significant psychological

and functional consequences. Functional deficit is related to the extent of surgery, the quality of reconstruction and the use of radiotherapy. Aggressive rehabilitation in speech and swallowing should ideally be instituted prior to treatment as part of a multidisciplinary approach.

Swallowing

Swallowing is a complex process and may be affected by tumour- or treatment-related damage to muscle, soft tissue or nerves. Surgical resection within the oral cavity, larynx or hypopharynx will inevitably result in varying degrees of impairment. The late effects of radiotherapy (see Head and neck cancer – 3) also have a detrimental effect. Swallowing dysfunction can be ameliorated by an exercise programme aimed at increasing muscle and tissue elasticity and maintaining range of movement in the jaw. Successful rehabilitation allows the patient to eat with relative normality, with reduced risk of aspiration. However, patients with particularly extensive surgery may never regain useful function, remaining dependent on a feeding tube (Fig. 3).

Speech

Resection of part of the larynx may affect the character, tone and intensity of speech, while total laryngectomy results in complete inability to speak. Commonly used methods of voice rehabilitation include the following:

- Artificial larynx – a battery-powered electronic device is used to create vibrations in the tissues of the neck. The sound is used to form words

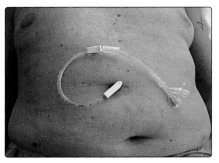

Fig. 3 **Percutaneous gastrostomy tube (PEG)** used during radical radiotherapy for head and neck cancer.

using movements similar to those required for normal speech production. Speech produced using this method has a mechanical sound.

- Oesophageal speech – air is drawn into the oesophagus and then expelled in a controlled manner to produce speech. This technique is difficult to learn, requiring intensive speech therapy and significant commitment on the part of the patient. A minority of laryngectomy patients use this method as their primary means of communication.

- Tracheo-oesophageal speech – a fistula is created between the trachea and the oesophagus, fitted with a one-way valve. When the tracheostomy is occluded, air is forced through the valve from the trachea into the oesophagus and can then be used to produce speech. The patient may occlude the tracheostomy using a finger or may be fitted with a prosthetic device which automatically occludes the tracheostomy in response to increased air flow in preparation for speech. This produces excellent quality speech while keeping the hands free.

Head and neck cancer – 2

- Cancer of the true vocal cords presents early with a change in the voice and is associated with an excellent treatment outcome.

- Advanced laryngeal and hypopharyngeal cancer may be treated with organ-preserving protocols using radiotherapy and chemotherapy, with surgery reserved for cases of treatment failure.

- Significant swallowing and speech deficits may occur as a result of cancer or as a consequence of treatment.

- Long-term enteral feeding may be required.

- Artificial means of speech include the artificial larynx, oesophageal speech and tracheo-oesophageal speech.

Head and neck cancer – 3

Nasal cavity and paranasal sinuses

Presenting symptoms

Symptoms are closely related to the anatomical location of disease. Tumours of the nasal cavity tend to present with nasal stuffiness and epistaxis. Similar symptoms occur with early lesions in the maxillary sinus. Lesions which extend beyond the sinus may produce swelling and numbness of the overlying cheek, proptosis and diplopia or swelling within the mouth at the alveolar margin or hard palate. Lymphadenopathy is rare.

Tumours within the ethmoid sinus frequently spread to the other ethmoid sinus and may infiltrate the bones of the nose, producing a swelling between the eyes. Extension into the anterior cranial fossa may occur but is often asymptomatic.

Management

The majority of cases present at a late stage and are treated with a combination of surgery and radiotherapy. Cases not amenable to surgery carry a poor prognosis as the control rates with radiotherapy alone are poor.

Surgery

Surgical procedures include lateral rhinotomy, rhinectomy, maxillectomy and craniofacial resection. Orbital exenteration may be required. These operations have obvious effects on appearance and function. Early rehabilitation and the use of prosthetic devices help the patient resume normal eating and speech as soon as possible. Maxillectomy creates a hole in the hard palate extending into the cavity of the sinus. This can be seen on looking into the patient's mouth. A maxillary obturator is a moulded prosthesis inserted through the mouth which corrects the deficit, allowing resumption of normal eating.

Radiotherapy

The tumour with a suitable margin added to allow for subclinical microscopic disease is included in the radiation field. Treatment of some normal structures will be unavoidable. Inserting a mouth bite will move the lower jaw out of the radiation field, reducing the dose to the oral cavity and tongue. The cervical lymph nodes do not need to be treated as the risk of occult metastatic disease is small.

Salivary glands

There is great variation in the treatment of salivary gland tumours, particularly those in the submandibular or sublingual glands owing to their rarity. In general, surgical excision of the lesion is the curative treatment. Adjuvant radiotherapy may be indicated if there is sizeable risk of recurrence.

Acinic cell carcinoma is a slow growing tumour which nevertheless has the potential for malignant spread. Adenoid cystic carcinoma spreads along the route of the facial nerve and characteristically displays a pattern of repeated recurrence after initial excision. Mucoepidermoid carcinoma may be of low or high grade with varying prognosis.

The parotid gland is divided into a superficial and deep lobe by the facial nerve. Facial nerve palsy is therefore a potential complication of tumour (Fig. 1) and of parotid surgery. The nerve is identified intraoperatively and the tumour resected while preserving the nerve if possible. A nerve graft is used if the facial nerve must be sacrificed. Incomplete excision, breach of the parotid capsule or metastatic involvement of the lymph nodes may be considered an indication for adjuvant radiotherapy.

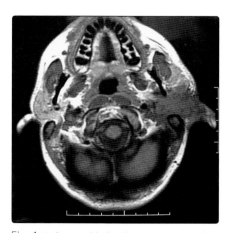

Fig. 1 **Left parotid gland tumour presenting with facial nerve palsy.**

Oral cavity

The majority of tumours in the oral cavity occur on the anterior two thirds of the tongue. Other sites include the floor of the mouth, the mucosa lining the cheeks, the gums and the hard palate. In general, early lesions can be treated with either radiotherapy or surgery. Small lesions have been treated using brachytherapy alone with high rates of local control reported. Larger lesions require external beam radiotherapy.

More advanced lesions require a combined approach. Locally advanced tumours will require extensive operations and result in significant tissue deficits. Reconstructive surgery using rotated muscle flaps or free flaps will be necessary to optimise functional and cosmetic results.

Head and neck radiotherapy

Immobilisation for head and neck radiotherapy

Careful radiotherapy planning will go to waste unless the patient's position on the treatment couch is accurately reproduced each day during treatment. Treatment of the head and neck region requires set-up accuracy within millimetres. To achieve this, a thermoplastic mask is used. This device (Fig. 2) is made for each patient individually and is fixed to the tabletop during treatment, preventing patient movement. The treatment machine is then aligned with marks made on the outside of the mask.

Side effects of radiotherapy

A high dose of radiation must be given to successfully treat the head and neck cancers discussed here. With many vital structures located in a small anatomical area it is inevitable that the administration of high dose radiation treatment in combination with chemotherapy will result in significant acute and late toxicity. Proactive management by an experienced multidisciplinary team can minimise the impact of mucositis and skin toxicity (Fig. 3). Late effects of radiotherapy are discussed below.

Cessation of smoking

It should be clearly explained to the patient that failure to give up

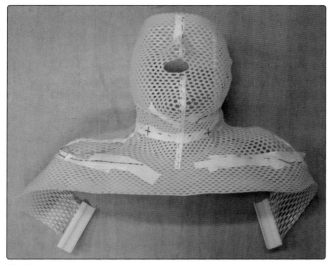

Fig. 2 **Thermoplastic mask used for immobilisation during head and neck radiotherapy treatment.**

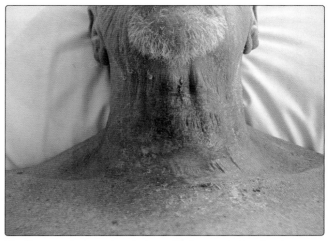

Fig. 3 **Acute skin reaction during radiotherapy for head and neck cancer.**

smoking will result in increased acute side effects and may compromise the outcome of treatment as well as exposing the patient to the risk of further primary cancers and cardiorespiratory morbidity. Every support possible should be provided to help the patient give up.

Late effects of radiotherapy

The long-term survivor of head and neck cancer may experience the late side effects of radiotherapy. These effects may be permanent, may not be amenable to treatment and may have a considerable unpleasant impact on quality of life.

Every effort is made during the planning phase to reduce the risk of late effects. Radiotherapy techniques such as intensity-modulated radiotherapy allow the high dose region to be shaped precisely to the shape of the tumour, however irregular, thus reducing the volume of normal tissue within the high dose area. This has been shown to reduce late effects, for instance allowing sparing of the parotid glands with a consequent reduction in long-term xerostomia. Late effects of radiotherapy are detailed here.

- Salivary glands – the parotid and submandibular glands are frequently included in radiation fields used to treat other primary sites within the head and neck. Inclusion in the high dose region results in irreversible damage to the glands and a permanent dry mouth (xerostomia) due to lack of saliva. The impact this has on a patient's quality of life varies very much from one patient to another. Some find the use of artificial saliva preparations useful. Most carry a bottle of water from which they constantly sip to keep the mouth moist.
- Soft tissues – fibrosis causes progressive hardening of these tissues, classically described as giving a 'woody' quality on examination. This can occasionally lead to difficulty in the diagnosis of recurrent tumour, which may present in a similar manner. Necrosis of soft tissues may occur after minimal trauma and may complicate attempts to biopsy suspicious areas. Fibrosis of muscles and soft tissues surrounding the temporomandibular joint causes trismus. Jaw exercises should be performed regularly to prevent trismus.

- Teeth – with the loss of the antibacterial functions of saliva there is an increased risk of dental caries and long-term care of the teeth becomes extremely important.
- Larynx – the character of the voice may be significantly changed in the short term due to oedema and in the long term due to fibrosis.
- Central nervous system:
  - Spinal cord – treatment is usually given in phases – phase I fields are the largest and usually incorporate the spinal cord. Phase II and III fields are smaller and are designed to avoid further treatment of the spinal cord which may be treated to 50 Gy with reasonable safety. Carefully planned radiotherapy should avoid ruinous late effects such as transverse myelopathy.
  - Cerebral necrosis – necrosis of the temporal lobe is a rare but potentially devastating complication of radiotherapy for nasopharyngeal carcinoma. Localised necrosis may be amenable to surgical resection.
- Bone – osteoradionecrosis is degeneration of the bone due to high dose radiation. Mild cases may present as a small area of exposed bone amenable to conservative treatment with debridement and antibiotics. More severe cases may require resection of the affected area with reconstruction of the subsequent deficit. The removal of unhealthy teeth prior to radiation treatment reduces the incidence of osteoradionecrosis in the mandible/maxilla.
- Eye – various structures within the eye may be at risk in the treatment of cancers within the nasopharynx, nasal cavity or sinuses.
- Thyroid – annual thyroid function tests should be performed to detect subclinical hypothyroidism, which may become apparent several years after treatment.

> ### Head and neck cancer – 3
>
> - Acute and late side effects of radiotherapy to the head and neck region are potentially severe.
> - Acute side effects include mucositis and skin reactions.
> - Late side effects depend on the structures included within the field – irradiation of the salivary glands may produce a permanently dry mouth.

Acute leukaemia

Leukaemias are a heterogeneous group of malignant haematological disorders broadly divided into acute and chronic. The acute type are characterised by a malignant clone of immature cells – they retain proliferative capacity but are unable to differentiate further. Acute leukaemia represents less than 1% of newly diagnosed cancers in the UK, with over 2800 new cases diagnosed annually.

Leukaemias are further divided into lymphoid, myeloid and biphenotypic subtypes. Morphology, histochemical staining, immunophenotyping, cytogenetics and molecular markers are used to define leukaemia subtype. Acute myeloid leukaemia (AML) represents 80% of adult leukaemias, whereas the most common type of childhood leukaemia is acute lymphoblastic leukaemia (ALL).

Aetiology

Leukaemia occurs as a result of a series of transformations that cause alterations in the chromosome and inappropriate expression of various oncogenes. Factors that increase the risk of developing leukaemia are outlined in Box 1.

Chemotherapy-related secondary leukaemias now represent 10–20% of all cases of AML; these are clinically and prognostically different from cases of spontaneous AML.

Adult acute myeloid leukaemia

Presentation

The incidence increases with increasing age. Patients may present signs or symptoms including:

- constitutional symptoms
- altered haematopoiesis
- splenomegaly (50%) (Fig. 1)

- skin involvement (10%) – violaceous raised non-tender plaques; chloromas are masses consisting of blasts
- hyperuricaemia related to the increased cell turnover predisposing to renal impairment
- spurious – hyperkalaemia due to potassium release from high white blood cell lysis during phlebotomy,

Box 1 Risk factors for leukaemia

- Toxins
  Radiation
  Benzene chemicals
  Drugs:
  alkylating agents: cyclophosphamide, chlorambucil, melphalan
  topoisomerase II inhibitors: anthracyclines, etoposide
- Congenital disorders
  Down's syndrome
  Fanconi's anaemia
  Klinefelter's syndrome
  Bloom's syndrome
  Ataxia telangiectasia
- Acquired disorders
  Polycythaemia
  Agnogenic myeloid metaplasia
  Myelodysplastic syndromes
  Aplastic anaemia
  Paroxysmal nocturnal haemoglobinuria

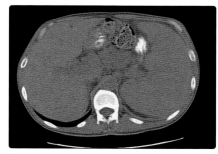

Fig. 1 **Splenomegaly.**

low glucose and arterial oxygen saturation
- hyperviscosity syndrome
- M3 variant may present with disseminated intravascular coagulation
- M4 variant may present with CNS disease
- M5 variant presents with tissue invasion such as gum hypertrophy.

Diagnosis

Diagnosis is established by examination of the blood film, bone marrow aspirate/biopsy and cytogenetics. The most important initial step is differentiation between AML and ALL; monoclonal antibodies that identify myeloid- and lymphoid-related antigens are of help. Auer bodies, reddish rod-like filaments of aggregated primary granules, are pathognomonic.

There are eight AML subtypes, each with certain characteristics (Table 1). Although the M3 variant only accounts for 5–10% of AML cases, it is distinguished from other variants by its distinctive morphology, younger patient age, specific chromosomal abnormality and coagulopathy. The chromosomal abnormality results in a PML-RARα fusion protein, which makes the cells exquisitely sensitive to all-*trans*-retinoic acid (ATRA).

The treatment of AML is divided into two phases – remission induction and post-induction consolidation or maintenance (Fig. 2). Cytosine arabinoside and anthracyclines are the two drugs most commonly used during induction, while the optimal post-induction consolidation regimen has yet to be defined. Allogeneic bone marrow transplantation (BMT) from HLA-matched donors in first remission has resulted in cure rates of 50–60%.

Table 1 Characteristics of AML subtypes

FAB type	Description	% of AML	Morphology	Cytogenetics	Prognosis
M0	Undifferentiated	3%	No Auer rod	Complex karyotypes, chr 5, 7, 8, 13	Poor
M1	Without maturation	15–20%	Rare Auer rod		
M2	With maturation	25–30%	Auer rods present	t(8;21) AML1-ETO fusion protein	Good
M3	Promyelocytic	5–10%	Auer rods numerous	t(15;17) PML-RARα chimeric protein	Good
M4	Myelomonocytic	20–25%	Auer rods present	Inv chr 16	Good
M5	Monoblastic/Monocytic	2–9%	No Auer rod		Poor
M6	Erythroleukaemia	3–5%	No Auer rods		Poor
M7	Megakaryoblastic	3–12%	No Auer rods		

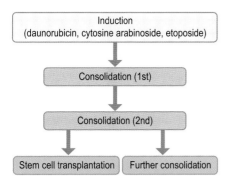

Induction
(daunorubicin, cytosine arabinoside, etoposide)

↓

Consolidation (1st)

↓

Consolidation (2nd)

↓   ↓

Stem cell transplantation | Further consolidation

Fig. 2 **Typical treatment plan for patients with acute myeloid leukaemia.**

Table 2 **ALL classification**				
Subtype	% Children	% Adults	Antigen expression	FAB classification
Early pre-B	55–65%	50–60%	CD19+, CD22+, CD79a+, CD10+, CD7−, CD3−, clg−, slg−	L1, L2
Pre-B	20–25%	15–25%	CD19+, CD22+, CD79a+, CD10+, CD7−, CD3−, clg+, slg−	L1, L2
B cell	2–3%	4–6%	CD19+, CD22+, CD79a+, CD10+, CD7−, CD3−, clg+, slg+	L3
T cell	10–15%	20–25%	CD19−, CD22−, CD79a−, CD10+, CD7+, CD3+, clg−, slg−	L1, L2

There are certain favourable features of AML:

- age <50 years
- de novo presentation
- white cell count (WCC) <10 000
- FAB M3, M4 myelomonocytic with abnormal eosinophils
- cytogenetics t(15;17), inv 16, or normal
- complete remission with one cycle.

Adult acute lymphoblastic leukaemia

This accounts for 20% of all adult acute leukaemias. Prognosis has improved in recent years, with remission rates of 60–80% and long-term survival of 25–40%. In 80% of cases the malignant cells are primitive B-cell leukaemias.

ALL is classified on the basis of both morphological and immunological studies (Table 2); the FAB (French-American-British) classification system separates it into three groups

- L1: seen most frequently in childhood; small homogeneous lymphoblasts (Fig. 3)
- L2: typical of adult ALL, larger more variable lymphoblasts
- L3: Burkitt's type, large vacuolated lymphoblasts.

The most frequent cytogenetic abnormality (20–30%) is the presence of the Philadelphia chromosome t(9;22); the *BCR-ABL* fusion gene results in a p190-kD protein product. Other abnormalities include t(8;14) and t(4;11). One third of patients have normal cytogenetics.

There are certain features associated with poor prognosis (Box 2). Treatment is based on regimens successful in children. Key factors in success are prolonged administration of chemotherapy (>18 months) and

Fig. 3 **Lymphoblastic cytology aspirated from an enlarged neck mass.**

routine CNS prophylaxis. Most patients have two cycles of induction chemotherapy, followed by intensification and prolonged consolidation. Allogeneic BMT in first remission remains controversial but should be considered for high-risk patients.

Biphenotypic leukaemia

These leukaemias co-express cell surface markers common to both forms of leukaemia; the categorisation is controversial – AML with lymphoid markers, ALL with myeloid markers, or acute undifferentiated leukaemia. These represent about 7% of all adult leukaemias. The complete remission rates are variable.

Childhood leukaemia

Acute leukaemia in children is very different from adult leukaemia. ALL is the most common malignancy in children and represents almost 75% of all leukaemias. Table 2 outlines the features defining ALL subclassifications.

In ALL the most common childhood subtype is L1 (85%); the remainder are either L2 (14%) or L3 (1%).

Most present with signs and symptoms of uncontrolled growth of leukaemic cells – fatigue, easy bruising and bone pain; 50–60% have hepatosplenomegaly or generalised lymphadenopathy.

Box 2 *Adverse prognostic factors in ALL*

- Male gender
- Age:
  children <1 year or >10 years
  adults >50 years
- WCC >15 000/mm³
- Prolonged time to remission (>4 weeks)
- Philadelphia chromosome positive
- Mixed lineage leukaemia (MLL)
- Elevated LDH
- Hypodiploidy (<45 chromosomes)

Secondary leukaemia

Usually secondary leukaemias are preceded by a variable period of anaemia, neutropenia or thrombocytopenia. The bone marrow demonstrates dysplastic changes in one or more cell lines. Platelets may be large and exhibit abnormal granulation; neutrophils may be hypogranular or agranular, with pseudo Pelger–Huet nuclei, and the red blood cells may be macrocytic with coarse basophilic stippling. Clonal, non-random, cytogenetic abnormalities involving chromosomes 7, 5 and 8 are found in 50–90% of patients.

Acute leukaemia

- Acute leukaemia is a heterogeneous group of diseases consisting of malignant proliferation of immature haematopoietic progenitor cells.
- It is divided into acute and chronic, myeloid and lymphoblastic.
- AML is the most common subtype in adults.
- Profoundly immune-depleting induction chemotherapy followed by prolonged maintenance therapy with CNS prophylaxis has good responses.

Chronic leukaemia

Chronic leukaemias may be divided into myeloid (CML) or lymphocytic (CLL). These leukaemias are characterised by a malignant clone of mature cells, which retain the capacity for differentiation in the early phases. Chronic leukaemias account for 1% of all newly diagnosed cancers in the UK, with about 3000 new cases annually.

Chronic myeloid leukaemia

CML is a myeloproliferative disorder characterised by an over-production of myeloid cells. It usually remains stable for many years (chronic phase) before transforming to overtly malignant disease (accelerated phase and blast crisis). A minority of patients (10–15%) may present in blast crisis. The median survival is 3–4 years; however, once the disease has progressed to blast crisis survival is measured in months.

The majority of CML cases (>95%) are characterised by the presence of a Philadelphia chromosome (Ph). This is a reciprocal translocation between the *ABL* proto-oncogene from chromosome 9 and the breakpoint cluster region (*BCR*) of chromosome 22; the fusion gene *BCR-ABL* produces a novel protein that differs from normal transcripts (Fig. 1). Philadelphia chromosome negative CML disease is atypical and follows a more aggressive course.

Risk factors for developing CML include increasing age, male sex, radiation or benzene exposure.

Presentation

The median age at presentation is 45 years. Patients may present with abnormal haematological parameters and constitutional symptoms. Some may present with abdominal fullness

related to massive splenomegaly. Rarely, markedly elevated white cell counts (>400 000/mm³) may cause hyperviscosity with blurred vision, respiratory distress or priapism.

Diagnosis

The hallmark of the disease is an elevated white cell count but the diagnosis involves examination of the peripheral blood, bone marrow and cytogenetics.

- Peripheral blood:
  □ leucocytosis (>100 000/mm³)
  □ presence of blasts
  □ left shift white cell differential
  □ anaemia
  □ thrombocytosis or thrombocytopenia.
- Bone marrow findings:
  □ increased cellularity, with raised myeloid : erythroid ratio
  □ presence of blasts
  □ basophilia
  □ reticulin fibrosis.
- Cytogenetics:
  □ Ph chromosome (95%)
  □ other chromosomal abnormalities include trisomy 8, isochromosome 17 or trisomy 19.

The blast percentage determines whether the disease is chronic or accelerated phase/blast crises. Table 1 demonstrates the haematological features. Uric acid levels may be high. The leucocyte alkaline phosphatase (LAP) score is low, reflecting qualitative neutrophil abnormalities, while the vitamin B_{12} level is usually markedly elevated.

Management

The approach to CML has changed recently; the standard non-transplant regimen for the initial treatment of all

phases has become the tyrosine kinase inhibitor, imatinib. Other approaches include interferon, hydroxycarbamide, busulfan and stem cell transplantation. Close monitoring of white cell counts, blood films and PCR allow for monitoring of disease response (Fig. 2).

Interferon is a second line agent for imatinib refractory, resistant or intolerant patients. It may result in haematological CR in 74% and complete cytogenetic response in 7–8%. Hydroxycarbamide is effective at reducing the peripheral malignant cell count and splenic size. It may result in 5-year survival rates of 45%.

Stem cell transplantation is the only curative therapy in patients with an HLA-matched sibling. Over 60% of patients have long-term disease-free survival after transplantation; the best responses are seen in those taken to transplant within a year of initial diagnosis. Relapse post transplant may be successfully treated with donor lymphocyte infusions (DLI).

Blast crisis is difficult to manage and should be treated as an acute leukaemia with intensive combination chemotherapy.

Chronic lymphocytic leukaemia

CLL is a clonal malignancy of B lymphocytes, or rarely T lymphocytes. It is clinically manifested by immunosuppression, bone marrow dysfunction and organ infiltration.

Presentation

It is a disease of the elderly with the median age of presentation 65 years, and peak incidence between 60 and 80 years of age. The male to female ratio is 2 : 1. Some may present with significant constitutional findings or recurrent infections. Over 75% of patients will have some lymphadenopathy at presentation (Fig. 3).

Anaemia may occur as a result of bone marrow infiltration, hyper-splenism or autoimmune haemolysis. Autoimmune thrombocytopenia may also occur. Although CLL tends to follow an indolent course, in 5% of cases an isolated lymph node transforms to an aggressive large cell lymphoma (Richter's transformation).

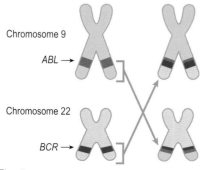

Fig. 1 **Philadelphia chromosome,** which is a reciprocal translocation t(9;22) (q34;q11).

Table 1 **Phases of CML**	
Phase	
Chronic	Blood/bone marrow blasts <15%
	Peripheral blood blasts and promyelocytes <30%
	Platelets >100 000/mm³
Accelerated	Blood/bone marrow blasts 15–30%
	Peripheral blood blasts and promyelocytes <30%
	Platelets ≤100 000/mm³
Blast crises	Blood/bone marrow blasts ≥30%
	MPO-positive
	TdT-positive
MPO, myeloperoxidase; TdT, terminal deoxynucleotidyl transferase.	

Diagnosis

It is characterised by an absolute lymphocytosis with a mature lymphocyte appearance. The malignant cells are CD5, CD23, CD19 and CD20 positive. Diffuse bone marrow involvement indicates a poor prognosis.

Other features with prognostic implications include:

- Cytogenetics: the most common abnormalities include deletion of 13q14, trisomy 12, deletion of 11q23 and *p53* mutations; the latter three are associated with poor prognosis.
- Somatic hypermutation: is a process where random mutations occur in the immunoglobulin heavy chain gene in response to B-cell antigen recognition in the secondary lymphoid tissues.
- Zap-70 is a protein tyrosine kinase involved in cell signalling which is associated with a poor prognosis.

Staging aids involve the extent of lymph node involvement and haematological function (Table 2).

Management

The majority of patients present with early stage disease; the median survival is 6 years. Table 3 details patient characteristics which affect prognosis. Indications for treatment include:

- disease-related constitutional symptoms
- bone marrow involvement with progressive anaemia or thrombocytopenia
- a lymphocyte doubling time <6 months
- recurrent bacterial infections
- autoimmune manifestations.

Treatment choices

Chlorambucil. An oral alkylating agent may be administered daily or in a monthly cycle. It is well tolerated.

Purine analogues. The most effective drug of this class in CLL is fludarabine, although it is more immunosuppressive, leading to increased infection risk. Combination with other agents (cyclophosphamide, rituximab or pentostatin) may result in responses in refractory disease.

Monoclonal antibodies. Alemtuzumab (anti-CD52) is effective in reducing both the peripheral blood malignant count and non-bulky visceral disease.

Corticosteroids. Have a direct lympholytic response and are effective for autoimmune cytopenias. Patients

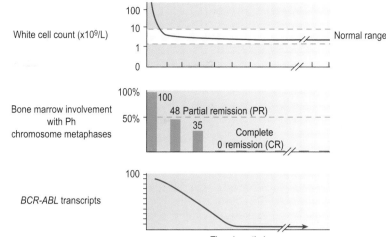

Fig. 2 **Treatment course in chronic myeloid leukaemia.** Patients continue with imatinib dosing as long as response is maintained.

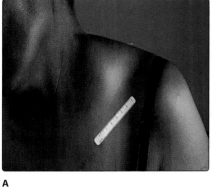

A

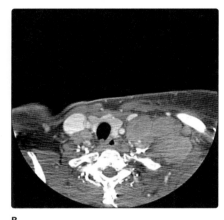

B

Fig. 3 **Lymphadenopathy** as found clinically in the supraclavicular area (A) and radiographically by CT (B).

Table 2 **CLL staging (Binet)**

Stage	Organ involvement	Haemoglobin	Platelets
A	≤2 areas	Normal	Normal
B	2–5 areas	LLN–10 g/dL	LLN–100 × 10⁹/L
C	Any number	<10 g/dL	<100 × 10⁹/L

LLN, lower limit of normal.

Table 3 **Prognostic factors in CLL**

	Good	Bad
Stage	Stage A	Stage B, C
Sex	Female	Male
Lymphocyte doubling	Slow	Rapid
Bone marrow appearance	Nodular	Diffuse
Zap-70 expression	Low	High
VH immunoglobulin genes	Hypermutated	Unmutated
CD38 expression	Negative	Positive
LDH	Normal	Elevated

with bone marrow failure can be treated with steroids until count recovery and then proceed to alternative therapies.

Radiation. May be used in the palliative setting for management of symptomatic isolated lesions.

Supportive care. Myelosuppression and infection remain the most significant complications of therapy in CLL. Prophylactic use of antibiotics in patients receiving combination therapy or fludarabine is recommended. Immunoglobulin replacement (400 mg/kg/month) intravenously reduces the risk of infection.

Chronic leukaemia

- CML is characterised by a markedly elevated white blood cell count and the presence of Philadelphia chromosome.

- Although allogeneic transplant is the only curative option, targeted therapy with imatinib results in superior survival for non-transplant candidates.

Plasma cell dyscrasias

Plasma cell dyscrasias represent a group of disorders characterised by clonal proliferation of plasma cells producing immunoglobulin. They include multiple myeloma (MM), monoclonal gammopathy of unknown significance (MGUS), plasmacytoma, Waldenstrom's macroglobulinaemia (WM) and amyloidosis. In general, these are diseases of the elderly, with their onset in the sixth and seventh decade of life. There are over 3500 new cases of multiple myeloma each year in the UK.

Monoclonal gammopathy of unknown significance (MGUS)

The distinction between MGUS and myeloma is extremely important when considering therapeutic intervention. MGUS is present in 3% of adults over 70 years. These patients have a paraprotein band which does not meet the diagnostic criteria for myeloma. One quarter of these patients when followed shall progress to overt malignant disease over 10–15 years.

Favourable prognostic factors include:

- immunoglobulin <2 g/dL
- no increase from diagnosis
- no decrease in normal immunoglobulin concentration
- absence of light chains from the urine
- normal haematocrit and serum albumin.

Multiple myeloma

The most important diagnostic finding in multiple myeloma is the demonstration of a monoclonal (M) protein in the serum and/or urine, found in 97% of patients (Fig. 1). The most common monoclonal protein is IgG, followed by IgA. Due to its pentamer structure, very high levels of the IgM paraprotein may cause hyperviscosity, while light chain accumulation may cause renal failure. Myeloma is characterised by bone destruction, bone marrow replacement and paraprotein formation.

Aetiology

The aetiology is unknown; however, risk factors include increasing age, sex, and environmental factors such as dioxins, benzene, organic solvents and ionising radiation. One study of bone marrow dendritic cells from MM patients found isolated infection with Kaposi's sarcoma-associated herpes virus (HHV8, human herpes virus 8), but subsequent reports have failed to confirm a pathogenic role of HHV8. The role of genetic factors is unknown.

Clinical presentation

Some patients are asymptomatic at diagnosis; otherwise bone pain, weakness and fatigue are the most common presentations. Bone pain occurs as a result of vertebral body collapse secondary to lytic lesions. Patients may be symptomatic from anaemia, renal failure or hypercalcaemia. Renal failure may be caused by light chain deposition, hypercalcaemia, amyloidosis, or related to NSAID ingestion for pain relief.

Myeloma patients are prone to recurrent infections due to bone marrow failure causing neutropenia, immunosuppressive effects of treatment and impaired antibody production.

Diagnosis and staging

The hallmark is the monoclonal spike on serum protein electrophoresis (SPEP) or urine (UPEP). Fifteen to twenty per cent will have no demonstrable paraprotein band in the serum but light chains will be found in the urine. Diagnostic criteria are outlined in Box 1.

Myeloma may be stratified according to β_2-microglubulin and albumin levels.

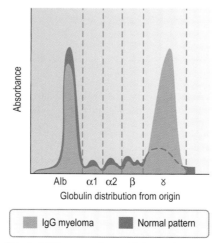

Fig. 1 **SPEP pattern in multiple myeloma patients** showing elevated γ-globulin region and reduction in other globulin fractions.

However, many other factors also have prognostic importance (Box 2).

Management

Myeloma management should consider:

1. control of the complications of the disease
2. control of the underlying disease.

Myeloma-associated renal failure is multifactorial; NSAID analgesia prescribing should be kept to a minimum and non-nephrotoxic medications considered such as

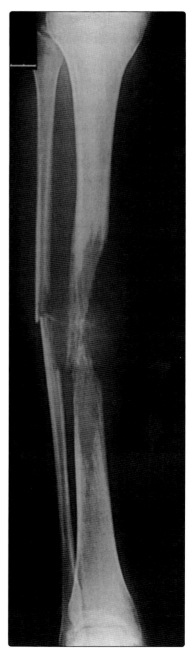

Fig. 2 **Lytic lesions of the tibia and fibula with associated fracture.**

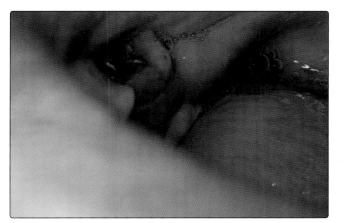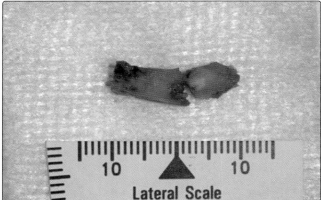

Fig. 3 **Bisphosphonate osteonecrosis of the jaw,** requiring surgical intervention.

Box 1 Diagnostic criteria for monoclonal gammopathies

Multiple myeloma
- Major criteria
  M protein; IgG >3.5 g/dL, IgA >2.0 g/dL
  Marrow plasmacytosis >30%
  Plasmacytoma
- Minor criteria
  Lytic bone lesions
  Marrow plasmacytosis 10–30%
  M protein less than the defined value
  Hypogammaglobulinaemia
- Diagnosis of MM requires one major and one minor criterion or three minor criteria

Smouldering myeloma
- Marrow plasmacytosis <30%
- M protein; IgG <7 g/dL, IgA <5 g/dL
- No or less than three bone lesions

MGUS
- M protein; IgG <3.5 g/dL, IgA <2.0 g/dL
- Urine light chains <1 g/24 h
- Marrow plasmacytosis <10%
- No lytic bone lesions

Box 2 Poor prognostic features for multiple myeloma

- High tumour burden
- Paraprotein >7 g/dL
- Multiple lytic bone lesions
- Anaemia <8.5 g/dL
- Hypercalcaemia
- β_2-microglubulin >5.5 µg/mL
- Albumin <3.5 g/dL

---

narcotics and paracetamol. Bisphosphonates are effective at controlling hypercalcaemia but also have an impact on the underlying disease by reducing skeletal complications (Fig. 2). Recently osteonecrosis of the jaw has been identified as a complication of chronic bisphosphonate therapy (Fig. 3). If bone pain is unresponsive to medications, radiation or surgical interventions may be required. Reversible causes of anaemia should be sought and may benefit from recombinant erythropoietin therapy.

It is important to determine if high dose therapy and transplantation may be possible in patients before initiating chemotherapy. When considering autografting, alkylating agents should be avoided until peripheral stem cell collection as these agents may prevent adequate collection at a later stage. Chemotherapy combinations such as VAD (vincristine/adriamycin/dexamethasone) are used for induction; if patients have disease that is responsive to 2–4 cycles of therapy, high dose therapy and autograft should be initiated. Allogeneic transplant has significantly more toxicity but may have more success.

Non-transplant candidates may be treated with a number of different agents. Melphalan and prednisone may result in an objective response in 51%, with median response duration of 18 months. Thalidomide alone or in combination is associated with significant responses, but these may be short-lived. The most common thalidomide toxicities include peripheral neuropathy, constipation and somnolence. Recently targeted therapy with proteasome inhibitors such as bortezomib have shown efficacy. Although interferon was traditionally used as maintenance, meta-analysis has shown little if any benefit to prolonged therapy.

Waldenstrom's macroglobulinaemia

This malignant disease of B cells appears to be a combination of lymphocytes and plasma cells producing an IgM paraprotein. The pentamer structure of IgM is responsible for its increased risk of hyperviscosity syndrome compared to other paraproteins. The median age of presentation is 65 years. Patients present with fatigue or symptoms of hyperviscosity. Purpura may be present. Classically these patients do not have lytic bone lesions or renal failure. Raynaud's phenomenon and peripheral vascular occlusions are associated with cryoglobulins.

Patients who present with marked hyperviscosity may require emergency plasmapheresis. Some indolent cases may be managed with chronic plasmapheresis while others require intermittent chemotherapy (cyclophosphamide, chlorambucil, fludarabine or cladribine).

Plasma cell dyscrasias

- Myeloma is a clonal proliferation of plasma cells.
- The combination of a monoclonal paraprotein and bone marrow involvement is essential for a diagnosis of myeloma.
- The median survival is 3 years; however, there is significant variation depending on risk factors.
- Immunocompromise is multifactorial.
- Treatment with a bisphosphonate is recommended to reduce skeletal complications.
- Stem cell transplantation may be curative in young patients.

Non-Hodgkin's lymphoma (NHL)

NHL is the seventh commonest malignancy in men and the sixth commonest in women in the UK. There are over 4000 new cases annually.

Classification

The classification of NHL has caused much confusion, with a reorganisation every few years. Clinicians have often subdivided lymphomas into low- and high-grade disease. Low-grade tumours are indolent, respond well to chemotherapy, but are rarely curable. High-grade tumours are aggressive malignancies needing urgent treatment, which if effective may be curable.

In 1994, the Revised American European Lymphoma (REAL) classification was widely accepted. The WHO classification is based on REAL, incorporating morphology, immunophenotyping, genetic and clinical findings. Approximately 85% of cases are B cell and the remaining 15% T cell (Table 1).

Aetiology

Risk factors include increasing age, male sex, prior radiotherapy, immuno-suppression and certain infections. Epstein–Barr virus (EBV), HIV, human T-cell lymphotrophic virus 1 (HTLV1) and *Helicobacter pylori* have all been associated with NHL.

Clinical presentation

The majority of patients present with lymphadenopathy or hepatosplenomegaly. Certain constitutional symptoms, known as 'B' symptoms, may be present in up to a quarter of patients – fever, night sweats, >10% weight loss. The most common extranodal site is bone marrow; however, other sites include the gastrointestinal tract, skin, brain, testis or thyroid.

Diagnosis and staging

Diagnosis is based on histological findings and cytogenetics. General morphology, immunophenotyping and genetic analysis are helpful. Clonality of B-cell lymphomas is confirmed by κ or λ light chain expression, while a clonal T-cell receptor gene rearrangement is diagnostic in T-cell lymphomas. DNA microarray remains a research tool.

Staging requires assessment with CT, bone marrow biopsy and lumbar puncture in high-risk cases such as bulky disease, bone marrow involvement or elevated LDH. The staging mechanism is the same as in Hodgkin's lymphoma. However, high-grade lymphomas may be risk stratified according to an international prognostic index (IPI), which helps management decisions (Table 2).

Management

Management is modified according to the underlying diagnosis, IPI and stage; the commoner lymphoma subtypes will be discussed.

Diffuse large B-cell lymphoma (DLBCL)

This is the most common high-grade lymphoma, usually presenting with rapidly enlarging lymph nodes (Fig. 1).

Stage I disease is generally treated with a combination of short course chemotherapy and radiation. The current standard of care is a combination of the monoclonal antibody against CD20 (R = rituximab) and CHOP chemotherapy (cyclophosphamide, doxorubicin, vincristine and prednisone).

Management of more advanced disease consists of 6–8 cycles of CHOP-R. Young patients with chemosensitive disease may be considered for high dose therapy followed by autologous stem cell transplant.

Follicular lymphoma

Follicular lymphoma is a common lymphoma characterised by the translocation t(14;18) and constitutive BCL-2 expression (Fig. 2). It follows a relatively indolent course with a median survival of approximately 10 years.

Treatment depends on the patient's condition and stage of the disease. A 'watch and wait' approach is not unreasonable in asymptomatic patients as early treatment is not associated with a survival benefit.

Treatment should be initiated for symptomatic patients, evidence of rapid disease progression, or significant visceral involvement. Combination chemotherapy is effective, resulting in durable response duration. Anthracyclines are generally reserved for use at a later time. Fludarabine is an effective salvage therapy, either alone or in combination with other agents. Monoclonal antibody therapy such as rituximab is effective with

---

Table 1 The WHO/REAL classification of non-Hodgkin's lymphoma

Precursor B-cell neoplasms	Precursor T-cell neoplasms
B-lymphoblastic leukaemia/lymphoma	T-cell lymphoblastic leukaemia/lymphoma
Mature (peripheral) B-cell neoplasms	**Mature (peripheral) T-cell neoplasms**
B-cell chronic lymphocytic leukaemia/small lymphocytic lymphoma	T-cell prolymphocytic leukaemia
B-cell prolymphocytic leukaemia	T-cell granular lymphocytic leukaemia
Lymphoplasmacytic lymphoma	Aggressive NK cell leukaemia
Splenic marginal zone B-cell lymphoma	Adult T-cell lymphoma/leukaemia (HTLV1+)
Hairy cell leukaemia	Extranodal NK/T-cell lymphoma, nasal type
Plasma cell myeloma/plasmacytoma	Enteropathy-type T-cell lymphoma
Extranodal marginal zone B-cell lymphoma of MALT type	Mycosis fungoides/Sezary syndrome
Mantle cell lymphoma	Anaplastic large cell lymphoma, cutaneous type
Follicular lymphoma	Peripheral T-cell lymphoma, unspecified
Nodal marginal zone B-cell lymphoma	Angioimmunoblastic T-cell lymphoma
Diffuse large B-cell lymphoma	Anaplastic large cell lymphoma, primary systemic type
Burkitt's lymphoma/leukaemia	
Primary effusion lymphoma	
Mediastinal large B-cell lymphoma	

Table 2 International prognostic index (IPI) for high-grade lymphoma

	Good, score = 0	Poor, score = 1
Age	<60 years	>60 years
Performance status	0/1	≥2
Stage	I or II	III or IV
Extranodal sites	0/1	≥2
Serum LDH	Normal	Elevated

The scores for each characteristic are added and the sum determines the prognostic risk group designation. Low risk 0–1, low intermediate risk 2, high intermediate risk 3, and high risk 4 or 5. Adapted from NEJM 1993;392:987.

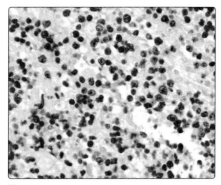

Fig. 1 **High MIB1 antibody expression** is a measure of significant proliferative capacity of the lymphoma.

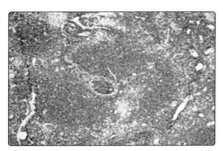

Fig. 2 **Lymph node biopsy** demonstrating grade II follicular non-Hodgkin's lymphoma with positive CD20 immunohistochemical staining.

minimal toxicity when administered alone; superior response rates are seen in combination with chemotherapy. More aggressive chemotherapy with stem cell transplantation should be considered in younger patients.

Mantle cell lymphoma (MCL)

This lymphoma is derived from the pre-germinal centre cells in the primary follicles and is characterised by a translocation of t(11;14) which results in cyclin D1 over-expression, which drives the cells through the cell cycle. Patients often have disseminated disease at presentation (Fig. 3). Anthracycline-based chemotherapy with or without rituximab may achieve complete remission; these responses are short-lived.

Burkitt's lymphoma

Two forms of Burkitt's lymphoma exist – the endemic type associated with EBV infection and a sporadic subtype that has no viral association. The disease is characterised by *MYC* over-expression due to a translocation t(8;14). Patients present with rapidly progressive disease. High dose combination chemotherapy is the treatment of choice for long-term responses.

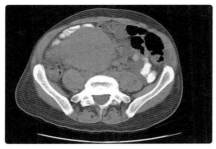

Fig. 3 **Disseminated disease at presentation** is not uncommon with mantle cell lymphoma. CT of the abdomen demonstrates a large intra-abdominal lymphoma mass.

Marginal zone lymphomas

These low-grade lymphomas generally present with extranodal disease. MALT (mucosa-associated lymphoid tissue) lymphomas may present with gastric or thyroid involvement. Gastric MALT lymphomas are associated with *H. pylori* infection and some may be managed with antimicrobials.

Peripheral T-cell lymphomas

This diverse collection of disease constitutes 6% of all non-Hodgkin's lymphoma. Despite treatment with chemotherapy, stage-adjusted prognosis is inferior to B-cell lymphomas.

Angioimmunoblastic T-cell lymphoma

This uncommon T-cell malignancy is characterised by lymphadenopathy, splenomegaly, skin rashes, autoimmune cytopenias and an IgG polyclonal gammopathy. Standard approaches include combination chemotherapy (CHOP), immuno-suppression or high dose steroids. Any observed response is short-lived.

Anaplastic large cell lymphoma (ALCL)

Primary cutaneous and primary systemic ALCL are distinct entities despite morphologically similar appearances. The cutaneous subtype is negative for the anaplastic lymphoma kinase (ALK) marker and generally presents with solitary lesions (Fig. 4). Occasionally these lesions may spontaneously regress or are associated with lengthy remissions.

Mycosis fungoides/Sezary syndrome

This is a disease of older patients who often present with patches, plaques,

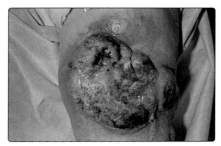

Fig. 4 **Anaplastic large cell lymphoma** may present with a solitary or multiple lesions in a single limb.

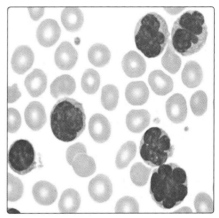

Fig. 5 **Blood smear demonstrating typical flower cell of ATLL.**

tumorous lesions or generalised erythroderma. Sezary syndrome is a constellation of erythroderma, lymphadenopathy and circulating malignant cells in the peripheral blood.

Adult T-cell leukaemia/lymphoma

Five per cent of human T-cell lymphotrophic virus type 1 carriers will develop ATLL. Patients present with lymphadenopathy, hepatospleno-megaly, hypercalcaemia, lytic bone lesions and elevated peripheral blood malignant cell counts with a characteristic flower-like appearance (Fig. 5). No effective standard therapy exists.

Non-Hodgkin's lymphoma

- NHL may be broadly divided according to cell type – almost 85% of which are B-cell and 15% T-cell.

- Clinically they are divided into low or high grade.

- Low-grade tumours are indolent, respond well to chemotherapy but are rarely curable.

- High-grade tumours are aggressive, needing urgent treatment, but may be cured.

- In general, T-cell lymphomas have a worse prognosis than B-cell lymphomas.

Hodgkin's lymphoma (HL)

Around 1500 people are diagnosed with Hodgkin's lymphoma annually, and it causes 300 cancer deaths each year. It represents less than 1% of all cancers diagnosed in the UK, with a slight male predominance. More than 75% of newly diagnosed patients are cured. Prognosis depends on many factors, including stage of disease and presence or absence of symptoms.

It has a bimodal distribution, one peak in early adulthood and a second over the age of 50.

Aetiology

Infectious agents such as Epstein–Barr virus (EBV) have been suggested as a possible aetiological factor as several viral latency genes are expressed in Hodgkin's lymphoma. Other infectious agents have been suggested but no conclusive evidence has been identified.

The development of HL has been associated with immunosuppression from HIV infection, transplantation or drug-induced. Some studies have suggested a genetic component; siblings appear to have a five-fold increased risk and siblings of the same gender have a nine-fold increased risk.

Pathology

Lymph nodes affected by HL consist of lymphocytes, histiocytes, eosinophils, plasma cells, fibroblasts and other cells. The mononuclear Hodgkin's cells and their polynucleated counterpart, the Reed–Sternberg (R-S) cells, which are the malignant portion of the disease, represent 0.1–1.0% of the entire cell population. Molecular studies have now identified that the R-S cell is of B-cell origin.

The WHO has divided Hodgkin's lymphoma into two groups – the majority of cases (95%) are described as classic HL and the remaining 5% as nodular lymphocyte predominant HL (NLPHD) (Table 1). L&H cells or popcorn cells are thought to be an R-S variant found in NLPHD.

Classic Hodgkin's lymphoma is further subclassified into four groups:

- nodular sclerosis 60–80%
- mixed cellularity 15–30%
- lymphocyte depleted 5–10%
- lymphocyte rich 5–10%.

The characteristic immunophenotype is positive for CD30 (Ki-1), CD15

(leu-M1), HLA-DR and CD25 (IL-2 receptor) (Fig. 1). HIV-related Hodgkin's lymphoma is almost universally EBV positive.

Clinical presentation

The majority of Hodgkin's lymphoma patients will present with painless lymphadenopathy. Lymph nodes are characteristically described as rubbery.

Neck or mediastinal lymph nodes will be enlarged in 60–80% of these patients; 10–20% of axillary nodes will be involved, while only 5–10% of inguinal nodes will be enlarged. Mediastinal adenopathy is an incidental radiographic finding in about two thirds of patients (Fig. 2). Hodgkin's disease tends to advance to adjacent lymph nodes in a contiguous fashion via lymphatics before becoming disseminated. Recurrent disease demonstrates non-contiguous spread and haematological distribution.

Lymphocyte-depleted subtype will often have abdominal nodal involvement and extranodal disease, while nodular lymphocyte-predominant Hodgkin's disease presents with localised peripheral disease often in the upper neck.

Hodgkin's disease may be associated with constitutional symptoms designated 'B' symptoms such as fever, night sweats and weight loss in over half the patients. The fever is known as 'Pel–Ebstein' and follows a characteristic waxing and waning pattern, becoming more severe and continuous over time. Night sweats may be drenching in 25% of patients. Pruritus, fatigue or alcohol-induced pain may also be seen in these patients.

Classic Hodgkin's disease may be associated with the development of other lymphomas, particularly B-cell type; the estimated risk of secondary DLBCL, Burkitt's or Burkitt's-like lymphoma is 1–5%.

Diagnosis and staging

Ideally an excision biopsy of a lymph node or site of disease is superior to a

Table 1 **Differences between classic Hodgkin's and NLPHD**		
Characteristics	**Classic Hodgkin's**	**NLPHD**
Pattern	Diffuse, interfollicular, nodular	Nodular
Tumour cells	Diagnostic R-S cells	Popcorn or L&H cells
Background	Lymphocytes, histiocytes, eosinophils, plasma cells	Lymphocytes, histiocytes
Fibrosis	Common	Rare
CD15	+	−
CD30	+	−
CD20	±	+
CD45	−	+
Epithelial membrane antigen (EMA)	−	+
EBV (in R-S cells)	+ (50%)	−
Background lymphocytes	T > B cells	B > T cells
CD57+ cells	−	+

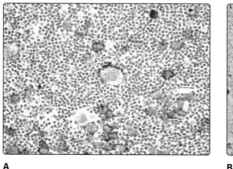 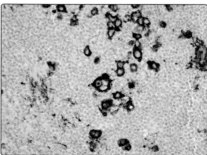

A   B

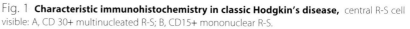

Fig. 1 **Characteristic immunohistochemistry in classic Hodgkin's disease,** central R-S cell visible: A, CD 30+ multinucleated R-S; B, CD15+ mononuclear R-S.

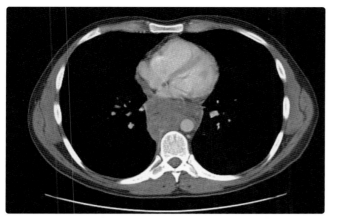

Fig. 2 **Mediastinal mass.**

Box 1 *Prognostic scoring system for Hodgkin's lymphoma*

Each positive response scores 1 point

Serum albumin <4 g/dL

Haemoglobin <10.5 g/dL

Male sex

Stage IV disease

White cell count >15 000/μL

Lymphocyte count <600/μL or 8% of total white cell count

Scores of 0–2 have an approximately 75% progression-free survival (PFS) at 5 years, while scores of 3 or higher have a PFS of 55%.

core or fine needle aspirate. An excisional biopsy allows accurate assessment of the pattern of growth, degree of cytological atypia, differentiation and presence of reactive components.

Standard staging includes:

- history for B symptoms
- chest X-ray
- CT scan of neck/chest/abdomen and pelvis
- Laboratory tests (complete blood count, ESR, liver function tests)
- bone marrow aspirate and biopsy.

The role of PET is currently being evaluated as a staging tool (Fig. 3).

Patients are staged according to the Ann Arbor Staging criteria, with the addition of the designation A or B, if the patient is without or with 'B' symptoms respectively:

- stage I: single nodal mass or extranodal site (E)
- stage II: two or more contiguous nodes on the same side of the diaphragm
- stage III: lymph nodes both sides of diaphragm
- stage IV: disseminated disease.

A prognostic scoring system incorporating stage, sex and laboratory values has been developed for advanced Hodgkin's lymphoma (Box 1). Mediastinal adenopathy is measured as a ratio of the transverse diameter of the thorax as seen on chest X-ray; it is known as massive mediastinal adenopathy if the ratio is greater than a third.

Management

In accordance with the European Society of Medical Oncologists

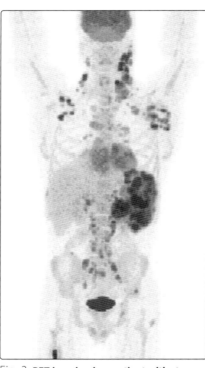

Fig. 3 **PET imaging in a patient with stage IV Hodgkin's lymphoma.**

(ESMO) guidelines, the management of HL depends on prognostic factors in addition to tumour stage.

Limited stage (stage I/II, no risk factors)

Recommend 2–4 cycles of ABVD (Adriamycin, bleomycin, vinblastine, dacarbazine; or an equivalent regimen) in combination with involved field radiotherapy.

Intermediate stage (stage I/II, risk factors)

Recommend 4 cycles of ABVD (or an equivalent regimen) in combination with involved field radiotherapy.

Advanced stage (stage III/IV)

Recommend 8 cycles of ABVD (or an equivalent regimen). Involved field radiotherapy should only be applied to bulky tumours (>7.5 cm) or to sites of residual disease.

Some cases of HL are left with residual fibrotic lesions. Therefore those with incomplete radiological response should be evaluated for active disease by biopsy or at least repeat imaging after an interval. PET imaging may be helpful.

After completion of therapy, patients should be followed every 3 months for 1 year, then every 6 months for 3 years and then annually. Thyroid-stimulating hormone should be monitored in all patients who received neck radiation. Breast cancer screening for women who received mediastinal radiation before the age of 25 years should start at 40 years.

Relapsed HL patients should receive salvage chemotherapy. If chemosensitivity is demonstrated, high dose chemotherapy and autologous transplantation should be considered.

Hodgkin's lymphoma

- HL is most common in adolescents and young adults, but with a second peak after age 50 years.
- It is a B-cell malignancy.
- Nodular sclerosis is the most common subtype.
- Accurate staging is the most important factor in determining management.

Paediatric oncology

The spectrum of paediatric malignant disease is quite different from adult malignancy. Leukaemia, lymphoma and primary central nervous system tumours predominate (Fig. 1). Renal tumours, soft tissue sarcomas (Fig. 2) and neuroblastoma account for the majority of the remainder. Carcinoma, the most common malignancy in adults, is very rare in childhood. Approximately 1700 children are diagnosed with cancer each year in the UK. Therapeutic advances over the last thirty years mean that 75% of children are now cured of their disease.

Paediatric oncologists face particular challenges. Delayed diagnosis is not uncommon in childhood cancers. Childhood cancers are extremely rare – a general practitioner will see few cases during his professional career and would require a high degree of clinical suspicion to make an early diagnosis. Variable presenting symptoms which may initially mimic common childhood illnesses compound diagnostic difficulties, increasing the risk of delayed diagnosis.

The therapeutic benefits of treatment must be weighed against the inevitable acute and long-term effects of treatment on the growth and development of the child. Children with cancer should be referred to specialist centres for treatment under the care of an experienced multidisciplinary team. The disruption of daily life should be minimised with efforts made to keep the child at home and in school as far as possible. Lifelong follow-up is necessary to document late effects of treatment.

There is a paucity of evidence from randomised controlled clinical trials regarding the management of rare childhood cancers. Results from single arm trials using historical cohorts as controls or from single institution studies are subject to many confounding factors and require careful interpretation. In this scenario, the optimal treatment plan is often under discussion, reinforcing the need for dedicated units in specialist centres with access to all treatment modalities. Treatment in specialised centres is associated with improved survival for conditions such as Wilms' tumour, discussed below.

Given the rarity of childhood cancer, advances in treatment can only be made by establishing cooperative multicentre trials. National and international organisations such as the International Society of Paediatric Oncology enhance communications between treating physicians, coordinate research endeavours and provide treatment protocols. The Children's Cancer and Leukaemia Group is a UK-based group which coordinates and participates in multinational trials in all areas of childhood cancer. This organisation and others also provide support for parents, siblings and survivors.

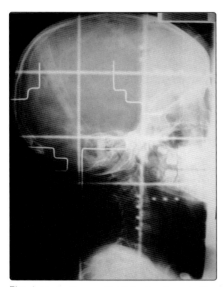

Fig. 1 **Radiotherapy field for treatment of the posterior fossa in a child with medulloblastoma.** (See p. 76.)

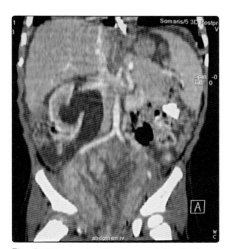

Fig. 2 **CT scan showing large abdominal rhabdomyosarcoma.**

Wilms' tumour

Wilms' tumour, also referred to as nephroblastoma, accounts for the majority of renal neoplasms in the paediatric population. The majority of children present with early stage disease and have an excellent chance of long-term survival. Wilms' tumours may be associated with rare genetic disorders such as Beckwith–Wiedemann syndrome in a small proportion of cases.

Pathology

Wilms' tumour may arise anywhere within the kidney. As the tumour grows, it displaces the normal kidney tissue, until only a narrow rim of tissue remains, stretched around the tumour. Classifying tumours as having favourable or unfavourable histology has been shown to predict long-term survival. Unfavourable histology includes the presence of anaplastic components, which may be localised or diffuse. The histological appearance is illustrated in Fig. 3. Up to 10% of Wilms' tumours affect both kidneys.

Various genetic abnormalities have been identified which are thought to produce Wilms' tumour including Wilms' tumour genes 1 and 2, both located on chromosome 11.

History and examination

The child typically presents with an asymptomatic abdominal mass noticed by the parents or picked up incidentally on examination. The mass may reach enormous dimensions and precipitate significant pressure symptoms such as nausea, vomiting and hypertension. Gross or microscopic haematuria may occur. The lungs and liver are typical sites of

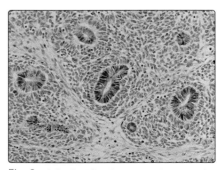

Fig. 3 **Biphasic Wilms' tumour.** Courtesy of Dr David Delaney.

metastases. Examination reveals a smooth or lobulated mass which is classically described as ballotable.

The main differential diagnosis is neuroblastoma, which can often be distinguished on the basis of clinical presentation. In general, children with neuroblastoma present at a younger age than those with Wilms' tumours and tend to be generally more unwell.

Diagnosis and staging

Ultrasound of the abdomen is easily performed and will establish that the tumour is arising from the kidney. It also defines the extent of the primary tumour and the involvement of local lymph nodes, and may identify lung or liver metastases. Tumour thrombus may be seen in the renal vein or the inferior vena cava. The other kidney should be assessed to rule out the possibility of bilateral disease. Children with genetic conditions associated with a predisposition to Wilms' tumour should be considered for regular renal ultrasounds as a screening test.

Full blood count, renal function tests and coagulation screen should be assessed in all patients at presentation. Urinary catecholamines are useful in that a positive test indicates neuroblastoma; however, a negative test does not rule out the diagnosis of neuroblastoma.

Imaging, surgical and pathological findings are combined to stage disease accurately.

Chest radiograph may be sufficient to detect lung metastases although CT is likely to be more sensitive. Thorough exploration at the time of surgery and meticulous pathological examination of the surgical specimen confirm the locoregional extent of disease.

The staging system most commonly used is that of the National Wilms' Tumour Study Group. This is based on the extent of disease and the completeness of resection of the primary tumour. Favourable or unfavourable histology is usually quoted in addition to the stage.

Biopsy

Traditionally it has been considered that performing a biopsy may increase the risk of disease recurrence. Performance of a biopsy has been included as part of the stage definition in the National Wilms' Tumour Study Group staging system, increasing the stage assignment for patients with localised disease that is completely resected. Oncologists may proceed to treatment on the basis of a clinical diagnosis, avoiding a biopsy, although the diagnosis may be incorrect in a small number of cases.

Kidney function

The function of the apparently normal kidney must be assessed prior to initiating treatment. Surgery, chemotherapy and radiotherapy all have the potential to impair renal function. Tools used to assess renal function include ultrasound appearance, intravenous pyelogram, renal function tests and DMSA scanning.

Management

Operable tumours are surgically removed. Neoadjuvant or adjuvant chemotherapy may also be given. Patients with more advanced stage disease may be treated with radiotherapy to the tumour bed in addition to surgery and chemotherapy.

Surgery

Operable disease is treated by complete nephrectomy and lymphadenectomy. Rigorous assessment and documentation of the locoregional extent of disease is performed as part of the surgical procedure. This information is crucial to accurate staging of the disease and to the planning of radiotherapy if indicated. Every effort is made to remove the tumour intact, without disrupting the renal capsule, avoiding spillage of tumour cells within the abdominal cavity.

Tumours which are considered too extensive for complete removal at presentation may be treated with neoadjuvant chemotherapy with a view to reducing tumour bulk, rendering the mass operable. This approach may also be used with bilateral kidney involvement to allow sparing of a portion of normal kidney tissue.

Chemotherapy

All patients should receive postoperative chemotherapy. Active agents include vincristine, actinomycin D and doxorubicin among others. Patients with more advanced disease are treated with more prolonged courses of chemotherapy.

Radiotherapy

Postoperative abdominal radiation may be administered to patients with advanced disease or to patients with early stage disease who have adverse features. The late side effects of radiation treatment have prompted research efforts aimed at reducing the proportion of patients treated with radiotherapy and reducing the dose given to those who require radiotherapy. The lung may also be irradiated in patients with pulmonary metastases.

Prognosis

The majority of patients with Wilms' tumour present with early stage disease and favourable histology and are cured. Advanced disease with unfavourable histology is associated with a much poorer outcome.

Paediatric oncology

- Leukaemia, lymphoma and primary brain tumours are the most common cancers in childhood.
- The majority of children with cancer are cured.
- The long-term side effects of cancer treatment in childhood are of increasing importance.
- Wilms' tumour arises in the kidney.
- Wilms' tumour is treated with surgery and chemotherapy; more advanced disease may also be treated with radiotherapy.

Primary central nervous system malignancy in children

Brain tumours are the commonest solid tumour in childhood. They include a wide spectrum of malignant and benign entities derived from various intracranial tissues. In contrast to adult brain tumours, most childhood brain tumours occur in the posterior fossa and typically present with raised intracranial pressure or cerebellar symptoms. The cause of most brain tumours in children is unknown.

The treatment of children with brain tumours presents many challenges. Radiotherapy in particular is associated with severe long-term morbidity in terms of cognitive impairment and endocrine deficiency. The younger the child at the time of treatment, the more likely it is that late effects will be significant. Clinical trials are now testing the hypothesis that chemotherapy can be used to defer or replace radiotherapy in certain situations. All children with primary brain tumours should be offered participation in clinical trials and treated in specialist institutions by a multidisciplinary team of experienced staff.

Medulloblastoma

Medulloblastoma is the commonest primary brain tumour of childhood. It arises in the cerebellum (Fig. 1), classically presenting with raised intracranial pressure and cerebellar signs. Typical cerebellar signs include nystagmus, ataxia (the patient tends to fall towards the side of the lesion), hypotonia, intention tremor and past-

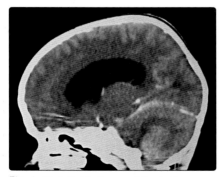

Fig. 1 **Medulloblastoma arising in the cerebellum of a 3-year-old child.** The ventricles are dilated, indicating hydrocephalus. Courtesy of Dr Jennifer Gilmore.

pointing. Midline cerebellar lesions characteristically cause truncal ataxia, abnormal speech and abnormal heel–toe walking. Initial medical management of raised intracranial pressure is outlined below. Preoperative insertion of a shunt to relieve intracranial pressure should be avoided unless vital as tumour seeding along the shunt has been documented. Decompression can be achieved at the time of radical surgery.

All patients should have magnetic resonance imaging (MRI) of the entire neuraxis (brain and spinal cord) performed to establish the extent of the disease as medulloblastoma may disseminate via the cerebrospinal fluid. Lumbar puncture is also indicated although it may have to be delayed until intracranial pressure is normalised.

Patients with operable tumours should undergo maximal resection. Adjuvant radiotherapy is given to reduce the risk of recurrence. The entire brain and spinal cord is treated to a dose of 30 to 36 Gy. The tumour bed or entire posterior fossa is given a boost dose, bringing the total dose to that area to 50 to 55 Gy.

Radiotherapy may be delayed and chemotherapy given instead in children less than 3 years of age to reduce the incidence of cognitive impairment later in life.

The prognosis for patients with medulloblastoma is improving. The majority of patients are now long-term survivors. However, learning disability is evident in the majority of survivors largely due to radiotherapy treatment.

Gliomas

Gliomas may arise in many locations throughout the brain. Lesions in different locations exhibit different behaviours and are associated with variable outcomes. Cerebellar astrocytomas are usually low-grade tumours. Ten-year survival rates of up to 90% can be achieved with complete surgical excision alone. Adjuvant radiotherapy may be considered when surgical excision is incomplete. High-grade lesions such as anaplastic astrocytoma (grade III) and

glioblastoma multiforme (grade IV) are less common and are associated with a poor prognosis. Chemotherapy may be beneficial for these lesions.

Brainstem glioma may be successfully treated when the lesion is low grade and amenable to surgical excision. Diffusely infiltrative, high-grade lesions (e.g. diffuse intrinsic pontine glioma) are not amenable to surgical resection and are associated with a median survival of less than 1 year.

Craniopharyngioma

Histologically a benign tumour, craniopharyngioma may nevertheless be associated with severe morbidity and shortened lifespan. Treatment may provide long-term survival but the majority of patients have a residual disability. Recurrent tumour is associated with a very poor prognosis.

Craniopharyngiomas usually arise in the suprasellar region. They typically present with headache, visual disturbance due to compression of the optic pathways or hormonal abnormalities. Visual loss is difficult to diagnose in a child and may go unnoticed until the deficit is quite marked.

CT or MR imaging typically reveals a cystic suprasellar lesion, classically containing calcified areas. A preoperative clinical diagnosis can be confirmed by histology at the time of surgery. Complete resections result in excellent long-term disease-free survival. However, aggressive surgery is associated with substantial morbidity. An alternative approach combines less radical surgery with focal radiotherapy. Abrupt deterioration in the clinical condition may be due to cystic enlargement or rupture within the tumour. Effective relief of symptoms can be achieved with drainage of fluid from the cyst.

Ependymoma

Most ependymomas arise in the posterior fossa. They may spread via the cerebrospinal fluid (CSF) and require MRI of the entire neuraxis as well as lumbar puncture to establish the extent of disease. Maximal surgical resection is associated with improved survival. Postoperative radiation therapy is usually given. Patients with no residual disease may receive radiotherapy to the tumour bed only, while those with more extensive disease will require treatment of the entire craniospine as described above for medulloblastoma. Radiotherapy should be done with three-dimensional conformal planning techniques to reduce the dose to normal tissues. The efficacy of chemotherapy for patients with disseminated disease and for very young children is under investigation.

Management of raised intracranial pressure

Headache which is worse in the mornings, exacerbated by coughing and sneezing and associated with nausea and vomiting is typical of raised intracranial pressure. Altered mental status may also occur. The sixth cranial nerve, which has a very long intracranial course, may be compromised, producing a false localising sign.

All patients presenting with acute raised intracranial pressure should have emergency imaging performed. CT may be preferred as it can be more rapidly acquired and is more widely available than MRI. This will usually identify the underlying cause. The following should be considered in the oncology setting:

- Space-occupying lesion:
  - □ malignant – primary or secondary lesion with associated peritumoral oedema
  - □ benign – haematoma or abscess may occur as a complication of tumour or treatment.
- High-grade gliomas may develop cystic areas. Rapid relief of raised intracranial pressure is obtained on drainage of the cystic area.
- Hydrocephalus – obstruction of CSF flow due to tumour results in dilated ventricles.

Tumour-related oedema will respond to medical management. Dexamethasone given as a 10 mg loading dose intravenously or by mouth and followed by 4 mg four times a day is started urgently. Improvement should be seen over 24 to 48 hours. If no response is seen, the dexamethasone dose can be increased, bearing in mind that very high doses and prolonged use of corticosteroids are associated with significant side

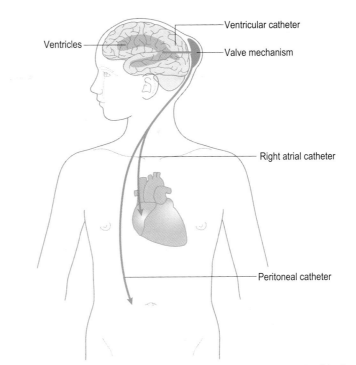

Fig. 2 **Intraventricular shunt.** Cerebrospinal fluid may drain into the right side of the heart or into the peritoneal cavity.

effects (Box 1). A proton pump inhibitor is given with dexamethasone to prevent gastritis and peptic ulcer formation in those with a history of peptic ulcer disease.

Mannitol is an osmotic diuretic which does not penetrate the blood–brain barrier. It creates an osmotic gradient reducing intracranial pressure as fluid is drawn out of the intracranial cavity. Mannitol is given intravenously in a 20% solution. A 100 mL dose may be repeated depending on response.

A ventricular shunt provides an outlet for obstructed CSF either to the atrium or to the peritoneal cavity (Fig. 2).

Management of seizures

Seizures may occur throughout the course of the illness; typically at presentation, postoperatively or at the time of disease progression. Standard anticonvulsant drugs are used. Monotherapy is preferred with blood

Box 1 Side effects of corticosteroids

- Gastritis, perforation
- Hyperglycaemia
- Fluid retention
- Weight gain
- Insomnia
- Proximal myopathy
- Mood disturbances, psychosis
- Immunosuppression
- Reduced skin elasticity, easy bruising, poor wound healing
- Cushingoid appearance

levels checked to ensure the therapeutic level is achieved. Additional agents can be added if monotherapy fails to control seizures. The use of prophylactic anticonvulsants in patients who do not present with seizures is not recommended. Prophylactic treatment may be used perioperatively. If no seizures occur these drugs should be discontinued.

Primary central nervous system malignancy in children

- Brain tumours are the commonest solid tumour of childhood.
- Medulloblastoma is the commonest brain tumour in children.
- Most childhood brain tumours arise in the posterior fossa and present with cerebellar symptoms and raised intracranial pressure.
- Curative treatment may be associated with severe long-term side effects such as cognitive impairment due to radiotherapy.
- The majority of children treated for medulloblastoma have some degree of learning disability.

Neuroblastoma and rhabdomyosarcoma

Neuroblastoma

Neuroblastoma is characterised by a broad spectrum of clinical presentation and biological behaviour with outcome ranging from spontaneous regression of disease to metastatic progression in spite of intensive treatment.

Pathology

These tumours are composed of small round cells arising from the sympathetic nervous system (Fig. 1). Specific genetic abnormalities within the tumour tissue such as amplification of the proto-oncogene MYC and the DNA content of the tumour cells correlate with survival outcomes. The degree of cellular differentiation and frequency of mitosis are also prognostic.

History and examination

This is a disease of infants and young children, with a median age at diagnosis of 2 years. Neuroblastoma may arise in any area of sympathetic nervous tissue, resulting in variable presenting symptoms depending on the location of the primary. The abdomen is the commonest site of origin (Fig. 2), with the adrenal glands

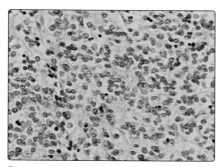

Fig. 1 **Neuroblastoma.** Courtesy of Dr David Delaney.

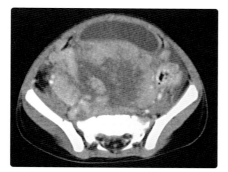

Fig. 2 **Large abdominal neuroblastoma seen on CT scan.** Courtesy of Dr Jennifer Gilmore.

and the abdominal sympathetic ganglia accounting for 65% of presentations. These children may be asymptomatic with the mass noticed by parents or discovered during examination for some other reason. Symptoms may include abdominal pain and pressure symptoms such as lower limb oedema secondary to lymphatic obstruction. Examination reveals a fixed, solid mass.

Tumours arising in the cervical sympathetic ganglia may present with Horner's syndrome. A paravertebral lesion may gain access to the spinal canal via the vertebral foramina, causing nerve root or spinal cord compression. Paraneoplastic conditions such as opsoclonus-myoclonus may occur. An affected child presents with chaotic eye movements and muscle jerks. Spread is via the lymphatic and haematogenous routes. The bone, bone marrow and liver are common sites of metastases. A child with metastatic disease may be quite unwell with associated fever and weight loss. The term 'racoon eyes' refers to the periorbital bruising associated with orbital metastases.

Investigations and staging

The evaluation of a child with suspected neuroblastoma should be undertaken in a specialised centre by a multidisciplinary team experienced in dealing with the condition. Biopsy of the tumour mass confirms the diagnosis. Staging investigations should include bone marrow aspirate and biopsy, CT or MRI imaging of the abdomen, pelvis and chest and radionuclide bone scan.

Neuroblastoma cells lack the ability to complete catecholamine synthesis, resulting in accumulation of intermediate products homovanillic acid (HVA), vanillylmandelic acid (VMA) and dopamine. HVA and VMA detected in the urine are useful as a diagnostic tool. Negative tests for HVA and VMA do not exclude neuroblastoma.

The International Neuroblastoma Staging System is used as the standard staging system. Disease is staged on the basis of patient age, operability of the primary tumour, lymph node involvement and the presence or absence of distant metastases.

Management

The intensity of treatment is based on the risk of progression and death from disease as predicted by proven prognostic factors including stage of disease, age of the patient, pathological characteristics, MYC amplification and DNA content of the tumour cells.

Patients less than one year of age with early stage disease have a very low risk of recurrence and may be treated with surgery alone. In fact, spontaneous regression of early disease is a well-documented phenomenon. Disease which is not immediately amenable to resection may be treated with chemotherapy initially.

More advanced disease with adverse prognostic factors is associated with an increasing risk of recurrence and mortality. Surgery and chemotherapy are standard therapy with increasingly intense chemotherapy regimens used with more advanced stages of disease. Disseminated disease, which is associated with very poor outcomes, may be treated with high dose chemotherapy and autologous haematopoietic stem cell rescue.

Radiotherapy to the tumour bed and the regional lymph nodes may help to reduce the risk of local recurrence in advanced disease although this is not definitely proven. Radiotherapy is indicated for incompletely resected disease and for tumour which progresses during chemotherapy.

Prognosis

Long-term disease-free survival in infants with early stage disease is in excess of 90%. Overall survival is even higher, as recurrence may be salvaged with further treatment. The prognosis for advanced disease, however, remains poor in spite of intensive therapy, with long-term survival in the region of 30%. Patients should be encouraged to participate in ongoing trials aimed at improving outcomes in this group.

Rhabdomyosarcoma

Soft tissue sarcomas, the majority of which are rhabdomyosarcomas, account for 5–10% of paediatric malignancies.

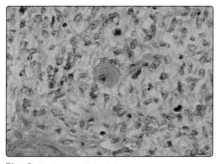

Fig. 3 **Embryonal rhabdomyosarcoma.** (rhabdomyoblast present in the centre of the field). Courtesy of Dr David Delaney.

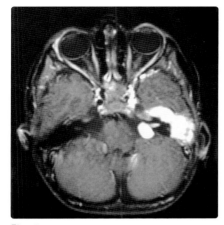

Fig. 4 **Rhabdomyosarcoma of the left middle ear seen on MRI scan.** Courtesy of Dr Jennifer Gilmore.

Pathology

Rhabdomyosarcoma is derived from the same developmental origin as skeletal muscle cells. Embryonal (Fig. 3) and alveolar are the two main pathological subtypes. Embryonal tumours are associated with a better prognosis than alveolar types. Distant metastases are present in one quarter of cases at the time of presentation and typically involve the lungs, bone and bone marrow.

History and examination

Rhabdomyosarcomas may occur almost anywhere. Symptoms are dependent on the site of the lesion and are therefore highly variable. The commonest primary site is the head and neck (Figs 4 and 5). Tumours arising in the orbit tend to present with proptosis. Lesions in the nasal cavity, paranasal sinuses and nasopharynx present with unilateral deafness or nasal stuffiness, which may present as mouth breathing in a child. A fixed, firm mass may occur in other locations. Additional characteristic primary sites include the extremities, genitourinary tract and thorax.

Clinical examination of the primary tumour must document the extent of

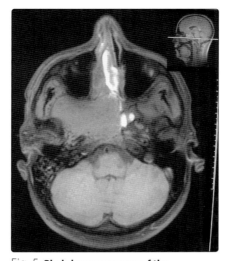

Fig. 5 **Rhabdomyosarcoma of the nasopharynx seen on MRI scan.** Courtesy of Dr Jennifer Gilmore.

disease prior to any intervention. Ideally, the surgeon, medical oncologist and radiation oncologist should all have the opportunity to examine the lesion prior to the start of treatment.

Diagnosis and staging

Biopsy of the primary lesion should be planned, with input from all specialists involved in the care of the patient. The specimen should be reviewed by an experienced pathologist as differentiation between rhabdomyosarcomas and other conditions such as the Ewing's sarcoma family of tumours can be problematic.

Routine laboratory tests should be performed on all patients. Either CT or MRI may be the preferred imaging modality depending on the primary site of the lesion. The associated lymphatic chains and the lungs should also be visualised. Radionuclide bone scan and bone marrow aspirate and biopsy determine bone and bone marrow involvement, respectively.

The Intergroup Rhabdomyosarcoma Study Group (IRSG) has defined a staging system based on the extent and resectability of the primary tumour.

Primary tumour site also has an impact on prognosis; for example, tumours arising within the orbit are associated with superior long-term outcomes when compared to other primary sites.

Management

Patients may be divided into low, intermediate and high risk groups based on prognostic factors described above, for the purposes of assigning treatment. Historically very poor outcomes were achieved with local treatments alone due to a high incidence of occult metastatic disease at the time of presentation. Outcome has substantially improved with the addition of multi-agent chemotherapy consisting of combinations of vincristine, dactinomycin and cyclophosphamide.

Resection of the primary tumour with a clear margin is the operation of choice. Sophisticated reconstructive and rehabilitation techniques may be required for lesions of the head and neck and extremities. If local radiotherapy is given to the primary site and the draining lymph nodes, late morbidity will be increased.

One treatment approach seeks to limit the toxicity of local therapies by treating with systemic chemotherapy initially, with a view to reducing tumour bulk and facilitating less radical surgery. Radiotherapy is reserved for patients with residual disease postoperatively or involvement of the lymph nodes. Alternatively, aggressive local therapy may be introduced early with a view to minimising the risk of local recurrence, while accepting the toxicity of therapy.

Prognosis

The majority of patients with localised disease are cured. Disseminated disease is associated with a long-term survival of approximately 30%.

Neuroblastoma and rhabdomyosarcoma

- Neuroblastoma arises from the sympathetic nervous system, most commonly within the abdomen.
- *MYC* amplification is associated with a poorer outcome in neuroblastoma.
- The majority of patients with early stage neuroblastoma are cured.
- Efforts to improve outcome in advanced stage neuroblastoma are ongoing.
- Rhabdomyosarcoma arises most commonly in the head and neck region.
- Surgery and chemotherapy are used in the treatment of rhabdomyosarcoma.
- Any additional benefit from radiotherapy must be weighed against increased toxicity.

Skin cancers

The incidence of skin cancer is rising in people of Caucasian descent due to increased sun exposure and an ageing population. Skin cancers are usually referred to as melanoma or non-melanoma cancers, the latter including basal cell carcinoma (BCC) and squamous cell carcinoma (SCC).

Epidemiology

Non-melanoma skin cancer is the most common cancer in humans with over 55 000 cases diagnosed per year in the UK. Most of these are BCCs. Malignant melanoma is much less common, with approximately 6000 cases per year diagnosed. The incidence increases with decreasing latitude. Worldwide the highest incidence of melanoma is in Australia. The melanin in skin affords protection, resulting in a lower incidence in those with darker skin colours.

Aetiology

The development of skin cancer depends on the interplay between environmental factors, the immune system and genetic predisposition.

Sun exposure

Exposure to ultraviolet light (sunlight) is a major risk factor for both melanoma and non-melanoma skin cancer. The popularity of sun holidays, outdoor recreation and the desirability of a year round tan have all resulted in lifestyles with an increased amount of sun exposure. Depletion of the ozone layer may also contribute. Malignant melanoma is known to be associated with sun exposure in childhood and with a history of severe sunburn; however, the mechanism of causation is not clear-cut as the disease may occur in locations not routinely exposed to the sun (Box 1). Fair-skinned people who do not tan are at increased risk of developing skin cancer.

Environmental agents

Ingestion of arsenic and phototherapy with psoralens for treatment of psoriasis are also associated with an increased risk of skin cancer.

Ionising radiation

Exposure to therapeutic or environmental ionising radiation has been associated with a higher incidence of skin cancers.

Genetic predisposition

Inherited conditions such as Gorlin's syndrome and xeroderma pigmentosum are associated with the development of multiple skin cancers. First degree relatives of melanoma sufferers have a higher incidence of the disease. The tumour suppressor gene CDKN2A accounts for up to one third of hereditary cases.

Immunosuppression

Patients who require long-term immunosuppression after solid organ transplant have a substantially increased risk of both SCC and BCC although SCC predominates. Lesions may occur in multiple sites and are more likely to recur after treatment.

Pathology

Basal cell carcinoma grows as islands of cells which form variable patterns within the connective tissue (Fig. 1). This gives rise to a variation in gross appearance with clinical subtypes including nodular, ulcerative, cystic,

---

Box 1 Site of skin cancer at presentation

Basal and squamous cell carcinoma
- Sun-exposed areas
- Head and neck
  - Behind the ear
  - Inner canthus
  - Eyelid
- Back of the hands
- Never affects palms, soles

Malignant melanoma
- Lower limb
- Trunk
- Head and neck
- May affect:
  - Palms
  - Soles
  - Mucosal surfaces
  - Nail bed
  - Retina
  - Other sites

---

superficial, pigmented and morphoeic. Morphoeic BCC is characterised by a depigmented fibrotic area of skin which makes delineation of the tumour borders difficult. Distant metastases are extremely uncommon.

Squamous cell carcinoma arises from the epithelial keratinocytes and shows a progression from dysplasia to invasive disease. Lesions confined to the epidermis are referred to as Bowen's disease. Sun damage frequently gives rise to actinic keratosis, a benign, red, scaly lesion which may ultimately harbour squamous cell carcinoma. SCC may metastasise to the regional lymph nodes or distant sites in 5% of cases.

Melanomas are derived from melanocytes. The commonest types of melanoma and their typical gross appearances are listed in Table 1. The maximal thickness of the tumour, first described by Breslow, correlates with survival and is part of the current staging system. Clark's level, which measures the histological depth of the tumour within the skin, is a less reliable indicator of prognosis. The histological appearance of melanoma

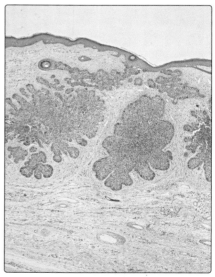

Fig. 1 **Basal cell carcinoma (×10).** Courtesy of Dr David Delaney.

Table 1 **Types of melanoma**		
Superficial spreading	70%	Dark area arising in pre-existing naevus, classically asymmetrical with variable colour
Nodular	20%	Dark nodule, uniform in colour, although may be amelanotic; majority arise in normal skin
Lentigo maligna melanoma	5%	Occurs on face and neck of older patients in areas of sun damage
Acral-lentiginous	5%	Palms and soles, subungual location

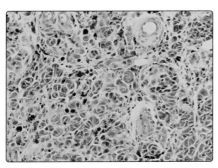

Fig. 2 **Malignant melanoma.** Courtesy of Dr David Delaney.

is illustrated in Fig. 2. Malignant melanoma may produce satellite nodules in the skin surrounding the primary lesion and spread to the regional lymph nodes. Distant metastases most commonly occur in the lungs, liver and brain.

History and examination

A classic BCC has a raised margin with a pearly appearance and telangiectasia although variations are common, as described above. Extensive ulceration and local destruction occurs if a lesion is neglected. The phrase 'rodent ulcer' may be used to describe this ulcerative appearance. BCC is usually associated with a history of slow progression over a period of years. SCC typically presents with an ulcerating lesion lacking the pearly raised margin of a BCC; however, the two may be indistinguishable clinically.

Melanomas are usually pigmented lesions, although non-pigmented melanomas also occur. Superficial spreading melanoma arises in a pre-existing pigmented lesion. The following new symptoms should be considered suspicious:

- increase in size
- change in colour
- asymmetry
- spontaneous bleeding
- inflammation
- itching.

The primary lesion should be examined to ascertain site, size and degree of fixity to the skin and surrounding structures. A thorough search for additional skin lesions should be carried out. The draining lymph nodes should be systematically examined.

Investigation and staging

A punch biopsy, done under local anaesthetic, is ideal for confirming the histological diagnosis of a BCC or SCC. If the clinical appearance is typical, excision biopsy will provide diagnosis

and treatment in one procedure. Enlarged lymph nodes may be assessed by fine needle aspiration. Staging investigations are indicated neither for BCCs nor for the majority of SCCs.

Suspected melanoma can be excised with a normal margin, with wider excision performed at a later date should melanoma be diagnosed on pathology. The regional lymph nodes can be assessed using sentinel lymph node techniques as described in the chapter on surgical oncology. Staging investigations should be performed for patients with node-positive malignant melanoma.

Management

Melanoma

The primary lesion

Curative treatment of a primary lesion consists of surgical excision with a suitable margin. The margin required is dependent on the thickness of the lesion, varying from 1–2 cm for lesions <2 mm thick to 3 cm for lesions >2 mm thick. Melanomas arising in particular locations require alternative surgical approaches; for example, subungual melanoma may be treated by amputation at the distal interphalangeal joint. Reconstructive procedures may also be required.

The lymph nodes

Metastatic disease in the regional lymph nodes is treated by complete dissection of the relevant nodal group. Patients with clinically negative nodes who are at high risk of occult metastases may undergo sentinel lymph node biopsy. A positive sentinel node biopsy should be followed by nodal dissection.

Adjuvant treatment

Adjuvant treatment for advanced or metastatic melanoma decreases recurrence rates and produces disease response but overall survival has not been significantly improved. Chemotherapy and immunotherapy have been used alone or in combination.

BCC and SCC

The preferred method of treatment depends on tumour site and size and local expertise. Most patients are

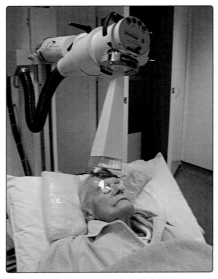

Fig. 3 **Radiotherapy treatment of a skin lesion.** Lead is used to shape the area treated by radiation and to protect sensitive structures such as the eyes.

treated by either surgery or radiotherapy. Local treatment results in cure rates of up to 90–95% in BCC and localised SCC. Postoperative radiotherapy may be given if complete surgical excision is not achieved.

- Surgery
  - excision ± reconstruction
  - Moh's microsurgery – successive levels of tissues are removed until clear margins are attained; a labour-intensive procedure not available to all patients.
- Radiotherapy – low energy photon beams or electrons are used to treat the superficial layers of the skin (Fig. 3). Long-term results are comparable to surgery.
- Cryotherapy.
- Topical 5-fluorouracil.

Metastatic SCC may be treated with systemic chemotherapy, although response rates are low and survival poor.

Prevention

Primary prevention measures are aimed at decreasing sun exposure. Liberally applied sun cream with a sun protection factor of at least 15, limited sun exposure between 10 a.m. and 4 p.m. and wearing protective clothes (e.g. long sleeves) form the basis of most sun protection advice.

Skin cancers

- The incidence of skin cancer is rising.
- Increased sun exposure is a major causative factor.
- Basal cell and squamous cell carcinomas are the most common cancers in humans.
- Surgery or radiotherapy for localised basal cell or squamous cell carcinoma produces high cure rates.
- Surgery forms the mainstay of treatment for malignant melanoma.

Endocrine cancer

This title encompasses a group of cancers that arise from hormone-producing endocrine tissue (Fig. 1). A group of inherited endocrine cancer syndromes are known as the multiple endocrine neoplasia (MEN) syndromes.

Thyroid cancer

Almost 1500 thyroid cancers are diagnosed in the UK each year, representing 1% of all cancers. The 5-year survival rate approaches 75%. It affects women three times more often than men, occurring between the ages of 25 and 65 years. Most cases are sporadic; however, 25% of medullary cancer cases have a familial association. The greatest risk factor is radiation exposure.

Four main subtypes exist, but they are often divided into two categories: well differentiated (papillary and follicular) and poorly differentiated (medullary and anaplastic):

- Papillary cancer is the commonest thyroid cancer (70%), presenting with multifocal disease and lymph node involvement (40%).

- Follicular cancer represents 15% of thyroid cancers; they may metastasise early to lung and bone.
- Medullary carcinoma (4%) arises from parafollicular cells and produces calcitonin. It is found in three hereditary syndromes – MEN 2A, MEN 2B and familial medullary thyroid cancer, all associated with mutations of the *RET* proto-oncogene.
- Anaplastic carcinoma (1–2%) is the most aggressive cancer, presenting in older patients with rapidly growing neck mass. The average survival is 3–6 months.

Ultrasound can be of benefit in distinguishing between cystic and solid lesions, but CT is superior for differentiating anatomy (Fig. 2). Once malignancy is confirmed, resectable patients proceed to either partial or complete thyroidectomy. Features associated with a good prognosis are outlined in Box 1.

Adjuvant radioiodine ablation should be considered in all follicular and papillary thyroid cancer patients, as it reduces local and distant recurrences.

External beam radiation may be considered for unresectable patients.

Parathyroid cancer

Parathyroid cancer is extremely rare, constituting less than 0.01% of all cancers and 5% of all parathyroid masses. The majority of parathyroid cancers are functional, with marked hypercalcaemia and hypophosphataemia. Fifty per cent of patients present with a neck mass.

Localisation studies including sestamibi scanning, ultrasound, MRI and CT, although performed, may be unhelpful in 30% of cases. A sestamibi scan is a radionuclide scan using technetium-99 to localise areas of overactive tissue within either the gland or metastatic disease. Selective venous catheterisation for parathyroid hormone may be of use in localising the tumour.

Primary therapy is surgical. The role for chemotherapy is limited; however, radiation may be of some use for unresectable local recurrences.

Pancreatic cancer

Tumours of the endocrine pancreas are rare. These are often described as APUDomas (amine precursor uptake and decarboxylation tumours). They are named according to the hormone

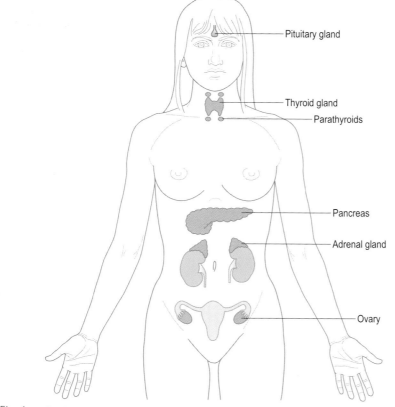

Fig. 1 **Endocrine glands at risk of malignant transformation.**

Pituitary gland

Thyroid gland
Parathyroids

Pancreas

Adrenal gland

Ovary

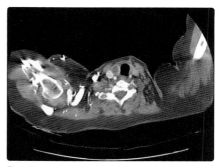

Fig. 2 **Cystic lesion right thyroid lobe.**

Box 1 *Good prognostic factors for thyroid cancer*

- Female sex
- Age <45 years
- Tumour <4 cm
- Negative surgical margins
- No extra-capsular spread
- No metastases

they produce and associated clinical syndrome.

- *Insulinoma* is the most common and presents in the fifth decade. Arising in the pancreatic β cells it is characterised by signs and symptoms of hypoglycaemia and elevated insulin levels. Measurement of pro-insulin and C-peptide levels excludes factitious hypoglycaemia as a cause. Ninety per cent are 2 cm or less in size, 10% may be multiple tumours and should raise suspicion for MEN. Fig. 3 demonstrates the histological features of insulinoma. Surgical resection is the only curative option. Systemic chemotherapy may have short-lived response rates of 50–60%.
- *Gastrinoma* presents in the fifth and sixth decade with gastric acid hypersecretion. Zollinger–Ellison syndrome is peptic ulcer disease, diarrhoea, oesophageal reflux and elevated fasting gastrin levels. Gastrinoma may be sporadic or familial, with 20–25% having MEN 1. They are found in the pancreas or duodenum, but frequently present with multiple tumours. Treatment consists initially of control of gastric hypersecretion with proton pump inhibitors and resection where possible.
- *Glucagonoma* may present with dermatitis, weight loss, diabetes and thromboembolic disease in the sixth or seventh decade. This cancer arises from the α cells of the pancreas. Eighty per cent are sporadic, 20% associated with MEN 1. Streptozocin or octreotide may be of benefit in controlling symptoms but with little objective response.
- *VIPoma* is characterised by Verner–Morrison syndrome of severe watery diarrhoea and hypokalaemia. It presents in the mid fifties with a female predominance. In the absence of metastatic disease surgical resection may result in cure.
- *Somatostatinoma* is the least common pancreatic islet cell tumour; 80–90% of patients have metastatic disease at presentation. Treatment consists of control of hyperglycaemia, nutritional support and surgical resection.

Adrenal cancer

Adrenal cancer is very rare; it represents less than 1% of all adrenal masses. The commonest malignancy is from the adrenal cortex.

Adrenal cortex tumours

This tumour is associated with a poor prognosis because only 30% are confined to the adrenal gland at presentation. It has a bimodal age distribution with a peak before 5 years and a second peak between 40 and 50 years. Over half are functional tumours producing hormones (Box 2). Most tumours are carcinomas, but anaplastic tumours do occur.

Radical surgery is the treatment of choice and when possible local recurrences also addressed surgically. Unresectable or widely disseminated tumours may be palliated with mitotane, systemic chemotherapy, or

> ### Box 2 Hormone-producing symptoms in functional adrenal tumours
>
> - Cushing's syndrome (hypercortisolism)
> - Adrenogenital syndrome
> - Virilisation
> - Feminisation
> - Precocious puberty
> - Hyperaldosteronism
> - Conn's syndrome (primary hyperaldosteronism)

radiation therapy. Unless a complete remission is achieved, a median survival of 9 months is seen with stage IV disease.

Adrenal medulla tumours

Phaeochromocytomas arise from the chromaffin cells within the medulla.

- 10% are malignant, 10% bilateral, 10% extra-adrenal and 10% familial.
- Episodic hypertension, palpitations, headache, sweating and anxiety are common.
- Radiolabelled MIBG scanning can identify extra-adrenal or metastatic disease, and at higher doses may have some therapeutic benefit.

Significant morbidity is associated with uncontrolled catecholamine secretion; therefore careful management is necessary. After alpha-adrenergic blockade has controlled symptoms, resection should be attempted for both primary and recurrent disease. Chemotherapy does not appear to have any impact on survival.

Carcinoid tumours

This slowly growing malignancy develops from neuroendocrine cells found in the small bowel, appendix, descending colon and lungs. Patients often present with advanced disease, typically with carcinoid syndrome. This syndrome of palpitations, facial flushing, diarrhoea, abdominal cramps and wheezing is due to the systemic secretion of serotonin, kinins, histamine and prostaglandins.

Surgical resection of the primary results in a 95% 5-year survival. Liver metastases may be amenable to local measures such as radiofrequency ablation or chemoembolisation. While octreotide results in symptomatic relief, the addition of immunotherapy (interferon) or chemotherapy can result in therapeutic responses.

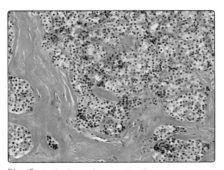

Fig. 3 **Pathology demonstrating an insulinoma.**

> ### Endocrine cancer
>
> - Thyroid cancer is the most frequent endocrine cancer in this uncommon group of cancers.
> - Most cases of thyroid cancer are functionally inactive.
> - Medullary thyroid cancer has a strong familial association.
> - Unless surgically resectable, the prognosis for medullary and anaplastic thyroid cancer is poor, unlike papillary and follicular cancer which are responsive to radioiodine ablation.

Primary central nervous system cancer in adults

Primary brain tumours are relatively rare, with approximately 4300 cases per year diagnosed in the UK. By their nature, however, brain tumours cause a disproportionate amount of morbidity and mortality. The diverse range of tissues within the brain may all give rise to malignant disease, creating various entities with significantly different natural histories and management requirements.

Metastatic lesions in the brain, which are far more common than primary lesions, are dealt with elsewhere. Certain benign lesions are discussed here as they may manifest in the same manner as malignant disease and often require similar management.

Epidemiology

Brain tumours have been recorded with increasing frequency over the last half century. The reason for this increase is unclear, although the increasingly widespread use of CT scanning and magnetic resonance imaging for diagnosis is partly responsible. The majority of primary brain lesions occur in adults >50 years of age.

Aetiology

Inherited conditions such as Li–Fraumeni and Turcot's syndromes among others are associated with an increased risk of brain tumours. Ionising radiation predisposes to the development of meningiomas and gliomas. This has been demonstrated on follow-up of children treated in the past for acute lymphocytic leukaemia or benign lesions such as tinea capitis.

Controversy exists over the role of various potential risk factors such as exposure to other types of radiation, head trauma or dietary constituents. Exposure to electromagnetic radiation from high voltage wires has been extensively studied in relation to incidence of childhood cancers, without conclusive proof of an association. Likewise there is no conclusive evidence that radiofrequency radiation emitted from devices such as mobile phones is linked with an increased risk of brain tumours.

Pathology

The WHO classification is the most commonly used system for categorising brain tumours. It incorporates histological type and grade. Histological grade is assigned on a scale of 1 to 4. Conventionally grades 1 and 2 are considered low-grade tumours, grades 3 and 4 are considered high-grade tumours. Histological grade has significant impact on tumour behaviour and prognosis.

The commonest adult tumour types are derived from the glial cells within the brain parenchyma. Collectively referred to as gliomas, these include tumours derived from astrocytes, oligodendrocytes and other cell types. Glioblastoma multiforme (grade 4) and anaplastic astrocytoma (grade 3) are high-grade astrocytomas. Low-grade astrocytomas include diffuse astrocytoma (which occurs in fibrillary, gemistocytic and protoplasmic variants), oligodendroglioma and juvenile pilocytic astrocytoma.

Heterogeneous tumours may contain discrete areas of high- and low-grade disease. A falsely low grade may be assigned due to sampling error. For this reason management decisions are made on the basis of histology, radiology and examination findings, not on the basis of histological grade alone.

History and examination

The symptoms produced by a primary brain lesion depend on the location of the lesion and the degree of oedema associated with it. Localising signs allow the clinician with a working knowledge of neuroanatomy to pinpoint the likely site of the lesion on the basis of the history and clinical examination. Classic localising signs are described in Table 1. Confusion, weakness, dysphasia, visual disturbances, headache and seizure are all common symptoms.

Tumour-related oedema may produce increased intracranial pressure classically presenting with headache which is worse in the mornings and associated with nausea and vomiting. Progressive impairment of consciousness and coma supervene without intervention. Ultimately the brainstem may herniate through the foramen magnum, an event referred to as coning.

The duration and progression of symptoms should be carefully noted. Rapid clinical deterioration is classically associated with high-grade lesions. The history should be obtained from both the patient and the family, who can often provide critical additional information, particularly in the presence of personality change and altered levels of consciousness. A full neurological examination with both positive and negative findings clearly annotated is essential.

Investigations

Investigations are purely diagnostic in the majority of cases. Staging investigations are not required as most primary brain tumours do not metastasise. Germ cell tumours and medulloblastomas may disseminate through the cerebrospinal fluid, but rarely metastasise to organs outside the neuraxis. Dominant prognostic factors commonly include histological type, histological grade, age and performance status.

Magnetic resonance imaging (MRI) of the brain with gadolinium enhancement provides excellent definition of the extent of tumour and surrounding oedema. Computed tomography (CT) scan with intravenous contrast is often adequate when MRI is contraindicated. MRI images of the brain and spinal cord should be obtained when CSF dissemination is a risk. The role of functional imaging with PET scanning is under investigation.

Table 1	**Examples of localising signs**
Location	**Signs**
Frontal lobe	Personality change, anosmia, leg weakness, urinary incontinence, gait apraxia, dysphasia
Parietal lobe	Dysphasia
	Gerstmann's syndrome occurs when the lesion is in the dominant parietal lobe – acalculia, agraphia, left–right disorientation, finger agnosia
Occipital lobe	Homonymous hemianopia
Temporal lobe	Dysphasia, memory loss
Cerebellum	Ataxia, intention tremor, nystagmus, hypotonia, abnormal speech, abnormal heel–toe walking

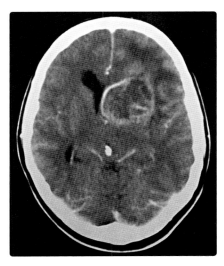

Fig. 1 **Glioblastoma multiforme on CT scan.** There is significant oedema, midline shift and rim enhancement.

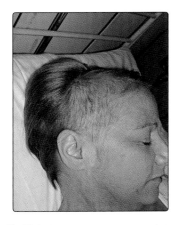

Fig. 2 **Clinical appearance post craniotomy.**

High-grade lesions typically enhance with contrast, are heterogeneous in appearance and are associated with significant surrounding oedema, which may produce a midline shift as illustrated in Fig. 1. Rim enhancement, also shown in Fig. 1, occurs as the active tumour grows outwards with a necrotic centre.

CT and MRI images are also used during stereotactic image-guided biopsy procedures to localise the biopsy site. Lesions such as those located in the brainstem may not be amenable to safe biopsy, in which case the diagnosis rests on clinical and radiological findings.

Management

Initial medical intervention is usually aimed at treating symptoms (see p. 77). This is followed by investigation and definitive treatment of the underlying primary disease. Treatment of intracranial malignancy is associated with significant morbidity. The degree of long-term impairment is dependent on patient, tumour and treatment characteristics. The risk–benefit ratio must be carefully considered and discussed with each patient individually.

High-grade glioma

Glioblastoma multiforme and anaplastic astrocytoma are associated with average median survival times in the absence of treatment of 3 months and 12 months, respectively. Surgery and radiotherapy form the basis of treatment. A small added benefit from chemotherapy may be seen in certain subgroups of patients.

Maximal surgical resection is the goal of operation. The postoperative clinical appearance is illustrated in Fig. 2. Maximal resection provides significant benefit in terms of symptom severity. This goal must be achieved without producing unacceptable neurological morbidity. The use of stereotactic mapping and intraoperative imaging may allow more precise definition of the target area, allowing improved resection. Craniotomy performed while the patient is conscious allows repeated assessment of neurological function, reducing the likelihood of damage to eloquent areas of the brain.

High-grade gliomas are highly infiltrative. Tumour cells have been demonstrated in oedematous tissue 2 cm beyond the evident tumour margin. For this reason surgery alone is unlikely to cure the disease and postoperative radiotherapy is a standard part of treatment even when resection is apparently complete. Three-dimensional conformal radiotherapy techniques allow delivery of a high dose to the target area while minimising dose to unaffected brain tissues. A typical dose of 60 Gy is delivered to the tumour or tumour bed with a suitable margin.

Temozolomide is orally administered and well tolerated. It has been shown to confer improved median survival in the treatment of glioblastoma multiforme when given with and after radiotherapy.

Low-grade glioma

In contrast to high-grade lesions, low-grade gliomas may demonstrate an indolent course over a period of many years. The majority of patients experience tumour progression after 5 to 10 years and will require treatment. Treatment options include surgical resection, radiotherapy and chemotherapy.

The timing of treatment remains controversial. The spectrum ranges from initial observation only to immediate surgery and postoperative radiotherapy with or without chemotherapy. In general, patients with a sizeable tumour and associated symptoms undergo initial surgical resection at the time of diagnosis. Radiotherapy may then be delayed until there is evidence of recurrent or progressive tumour growth, transformation to a high-grade lesion or symptoms such as uncontrolled seizures. Comparison of immediate versus postoperative radiotherapy has shown no difference in overall survival.

Oligodendrogliomas in particular have demonstrated encouraging responses to chemotherapy.

Pituitary adenoma

Pituitary tumours are most commonly benign adenomas. Symptoms are related to localised pressure, the production of excess hormones or reduced hormone production due to pituitary dysfunction. Baseline endocrine tests should be performed prior to intervention. Surgical resection may be accomplished via the transphenoidal or transfrontal routes. Adjuvant radiotherapy is indicated for residual disease although the timing is controversial. Some authorities advocate close observation with intervention at the time of tumour progression.

Meningioma

Meningiomas are usually solitary lesions arising in the meninges. The majority are WHO grade 1 lesions on biopsy. Approximately 70% of patients are disease-free 15 years after surgical resection. Postoperative radiotherapy is largely reserved for recurrent or progressive disease although adjuvant treatment may be given in the case of aggressive histological grade.

> ### Primary central nervous system malignancy in adults
>
> - Primary brain tumours are rare but account for a disproportionate amount of morbidity and mortality.
>
> - There is a wide variety of histological types with varying prognosis and management requirements.
>
> - The WHO classification of histological type and grade is commonly used.
>
> - Gliomas are the commonest histological type in adults.
>
> - Surgery with or without adjuvant radiotherapy forms the basis of management, with chemotherapy given in specific situations.

Primary bone cancer

Primary bone cancer occurs predominantly in children and adolescents. Osteosarcoma, Ewing's family of tumours (EFT) and chondrosarcoma account for the majority of cases. Historically, patients undergoing resection of the primary tumour had a high failure rate due to the development of distant metastases. Survival rates have been significantly improved with the addition of chemotherapy regimens aimed at controlling occult metastatic disease. The majority of patients with localised disease and up to 20% of patients with metastatic disease can achieve long-term disease-free survival.

Epidemiology
EFT and osteosarcoma show a peak in incidence in young adolescents. Osteosarcoma, which is associated with Paget's disease, also shows an increased incidence in those aged >65 years. These conditions are more common in males than females.

History and examination
Primary tumours of the bone typically present with localised pain and swelling in characteristic locations (Table 1). The anatomy of a long bone is represented in Fig. 1. Osteosarcoma is described as causing pain which is continuous and worse at night and is associated with reduced range of movement in the adjacent joint. Pain in children and adolescents is often attributed to injury or sporting activities and may be present for many weeks before the patient attends his doctor. A general practitioner may see only one case in her professional lifetime, a factor which diminishes the likelihood of early diagnosis. The finding of swelling on examination usually prompts plain radiograph of the affected area.

Clinical examination should define the site and size of the lesion and assess invasion of adjacent structures such as the skin, muscle, nerves and blood vessels. Typical findings are of a tender mass attached to the underlying bone. The severity of associated loss of function should be noted.

Distant metastases are present in up to 25% of patients at the time of presentation, most commonly involving the lungs, bone and bone marrow. Metastatic disease may be associated with systemic symptoms such as fever, fatigue and weight loss. Spread to the lymph nodes is unusual.

Investigations and staging
A radiographic work-up is completed prior to biopsy to define the extent of disease and to help the surgeon choose the optimal biopsy route. All imaging and histology slides are subsequently reviewed by the multidisciplinary team. Good interdisciplinary communication is vital; a diagnosis may rely on correlation of the pathology and radiographic findings, and local treatment decisions require detailed discussion of the relative merits of radiotherapy and surgery.

There are no universally accepted staging systems for primary bone cancer. Various systems have been employed in specialist institutions. These incorporate the known prognostic factors, which include:

- tumour size – larger tumours are associated with a poorer prognosis
- presence of distant metastases – metastatic disease is associated with a poorer prognosis; bone metastases confer a worse outlook than pulmonary metastases alone
- response to induction chemotherapy – extensive necrosis on histological examination of the surgical specimen after induction chemotherapy is associated with improved outcome

Table 1 **Clinical characteristics of osteosarcoma and Ewing's family of tumours**	
Ewing's family of tumours (EFT)	**Osteosarcoma**
Occur in young adults	Peak in adolescence and in those aged >65 years
Commonest sites include femur, tibia, fibula, pelvis, humerus	Typically located in the long bones of the extremities – occurs at the knee (distal femur, upper tibia) and the shoulder (proximal humerus)
Extraosseous location in 25%	Extraosseous location rare unless occurring in an area previously exposed to ionising radiation
Classically affects diaphysis	Classically affects metaphysis/epiphysis
Onion skin or moth-eaten appearance on plain radiograph	Codman's triangle on plain radiograph

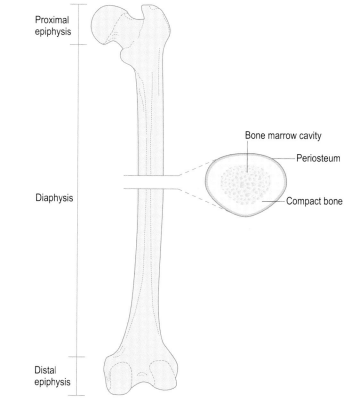

Fig. 1 **Anatomy of a long bone.**

Proximal epiphysis

Diaphysis

Distal epiphysis

Bone marrow cavity

Periosteum

Compact bone

- histological grade – high-grade osteosarcoma has a worse outcome than low-grade osteosarcoma
- local extent of primary lesion.

Imaging

- A plain radiograph of the affected area frequently raises suspicions regarding the diagnosis.
- Radioisotope bone scan will demonstrate a hotspot at the site of the primary lesion and may reveal bone metastases.
- MRI is the modality of choice for delineating the extent of the tumour within the bone and the surrounding soft tissue because it provides the best differentiation between tumour and normal tissue.
- CT scan of the thorax – lung metastases are the commonest site of metastatic disease and are best demonstrated on CT scan.
- Bone marrow aspirate and biopsy will identify metastatic disease.

Biopsy

Tissue samples may be obtained by core needle biopsy under image guidance or by incisional techniques. Ideally the surgeon performing the definitive resection should plan and perform the biopsy. The biopsy track and surgical drain sites must be excised en bloc with the primary lesion to minimise the risk of recurrence. Poor placement of the biopsy track or surgical drains may compromise limb-sparing surgery, resulting in unnecessary amputation. Poor placement may also influence the histology result if a non-representative area of an inhomogeneous tumour is biopsied.

Ewing's family of tumours

The Ewing's family of tumours includes Ewing's tumour of bone, extraosseous Ewing's tumour and primitive neuroectodermal tumours (PNET). Most of these tumours demonstrate a characteristic translocation between chromosomes 22 and 11 which helps to distinguish them from the other small round cell tumours of childhood such as neuroblastoma, rhabdomyosarcoma and lymphoma.

Management

Systemic chemotherapy

Localised disease is treated with induction chemotherapy followed by surgery with subsequent further chemotherapy. Induction chemotherapy may allow less extensive surgery by shrinking the tumour, treats occult metastatic disease immediately and provides powerful prognostic information in terms of histological response. Multi-agent regimens include active agents such as vincristine, doxorubicin, cyclophosphamide, ifosfamide and etoposide.

Local therapy

The primary lesion may be treated with either surgery or radiotherapy. Decisions must be made on a case-by-case basis to maximise tumour control and long-term function. Lesions that are considered resectable are usually surgically removed. Adjuvant radiotherapy may be given where there is residual disease or a positive margin after surgery. Some aspects of sarcoma surgery are discussed below.

The late effects of radiotherapy, in particular the risk of second malignancy when treating a young patient, must be taken into consideration when choosing to treat. The radiotherapy treatment field may include the entire affected bone and must at least encompass the tumour bulk present prior to chemotherapy. This usually results in large treatment fields, which combined with the need for a relatively high dose introduces a significant risk of late effects.

Osteosarcoma

The cause of most osteosarcomas remains unidentified but the following risk factors are known to be associated with an increased incidence of the disease:

- exposure to ionising radiation – proven link with subsequent development of osteosarcoma over a latent period of 10 to 20 years
- the use of alkylating chemotherapy agents
- Paget's disease
- genetic conditions – hereditary retinoblastoma and the Li–Fraumeni syndrome.

Management

Systemic chemotherapy

Treatment follows a similar pattern to that for EFT, with induction chemotherapy given prior to local treatment, which is followed by further chemotherapy. Chemotherapy regimens include agents such as doxorubicin, cisplatin, ifosfamide and high-dose methotrexate. All patients should be encouraged to participate in clinical trials aimed at identifying the optimal chemotherapy regimen.

Local therapy

Surgical excision results in acceptable local control rates and is the preferred option for local therapy given that osteosarcoma is considered relatively resistant to radiation treatment. The use of adjuvant radiotherapy varies from institution to institution. Radiotherapy may be given in the case of a positive margin to try and reduce the risk of recurrence.

Surgery

The aim of surgery is complete excision of the primary lesion with a suitable margin to achieve local control. Historically, amputation was routinely performed for lesions of the extremities. Advances in surgical technique and the development of increasingly sophisticated prosthetic materials have facilitated increasing use of limb-sparing surgery. While functional outcome is important, the oncological outcome is paramount and patients must be chosen carefully for limb-sparing surgery given that a wide margin on the primary lesion is required.

Reconstructive techniques involve the use of grafts and metal prostheses. Achieving equal limb length in a growing child presents particular difficulties. Prosthetic devices which can be gradually lengthened are available. A major disadvantage is that an operation is required to adjust the length of the device. Prosthetic devices placed at a young age will have to be completely replaced during the lifetime of a survivor.

Primary bone cancer

- Primary bone cancer occurs predominantly in children and adolescents.
- Osteosarcoma, Ewing's family of tumours (EFT) and chondrosarcoma account for the majority of cases.
- These cancers should be treated by a multidisciplinary team with experience in their management.
- The biopsy site should be carefully placed so that it can be completely excised at the time of definitive surgery.

Carcinoma of unknown primary (CUP)

In spite of the advances in medical imaging and laboratory investigations, a primary may not be identified in 3–5% of patients presenting with metastatic disease. It is defined as a cancer where, in spite of tumour biopsy, a thorough history, complete physical examination that includes head and neck, rectal, pelvic and breast examinations, chest X-rays, a complete blood cell count, urinalysis and an examination of the stool for occult blood, the source of the cancer is not identified.

This group follows an aggressive course with 1- and 5-year survival rates of 25% and 10%, respectively. The median survival for those with CUP is 3–4 months.

Significant improvements in immunohistochemical analysis have provided more accurate predictions of chemotherapy responsiveness.

Clinical presentation

The presenting features depend on the site of tumour involvement. Large studies have identified lung and pancreas as the most common carcinomas presenting as CUP, but other sources include breast, colorectal and prostate cancers.

The pattern of metastases may help to identify the primary.

- Lung metastases are twice as common in primary sites above the diaphragm than below.
- Liver metastases are more common from primaries below the diaphragm.
- Ovarian, GI tract and pancreatic cancers may present with peritoneal deposits.

- The site of localised adenopathy may suggest the primary, e.g. axillary – breast, lung or melanoma, high cervical – head and neck, thyroid or lung.

Pathology

Light microscopy divides CUP into five broad categories:

- adenocarcinoma (50%)
- poorly differentiated carcinoma (20–30%)
- squamous cell carcinoma (10–15%)
- undifferentiated neoplasm (5%)
- neuroendocrine carcinoma (<5%).

Adequate tissue is essential for performing immunohistochemical (IHC) analysis to clarify pathology further (Fig. 1). Different surface markers characterise different cell types, with certain markers present in epithelial tumours, others in lymphoid tumours, and still others in melanomas. The keratin family is a group of proteins that are relatively tissue specific, and examination of differential staining may be helpful (Tables 1 and 2).

Electron microscopy can be helpful in patients with poorly differentiated neoplasms. Certain cancers have characteristic appearances such as squamous cell carcinomas, melanoma and mesothelioma.

The use of DNA microarray technologies (Fig. 2) has been demonstrated to identify characteristic patterns of various adenocarcinomas and lymphomas and may aid in diagnosis.

Diagnosis and staging

Evaluation should include a thorough history and physical examination (including pelvic examination of women and prostate examination in males), complete blood count, serum chemistries, urinalysis, chest X-ray, and CT of abdomen and pelvis. CT imaging will identify exact sites of disease (Fig. 3).

- Presentation with neck adenopathy requires a meticulous examination of the head and neck area.
- Those with isolated axillary metastases most commonly have lung or breast cancer primaries. Mammogram should be considered in a female with adenocarcinoma.
- Squamous cell carcinoma inguinal metastases may be of genital or anal/rectal origin; therefore organ-specific investigations may be warranted.
- Serum beta-human chorionic gonadotrophin (βHCG), alpha-fetoprotein (AFP) and prostate specific antigen (PSA) are useful to exclude potentially curable extragonadal germ cell tumours and metastatic prostate cancer.
- Common tumour markers (CEA, CA19–9, CA15–3) are generally not helpful as diagnostic or prognostic tools; however, they may be useful to follow response to therapy.

Endoscopy such as gastroscopy, colonoscopy or bronchoscopy should be directed towards investigating specific complaints. Extent of further investigations depends on the attending physician; however, exhaustive searches are of benefit in less than 20% of cases of CUP. But it is

Table 1 **Immunohistochemical studies**	
Tumour type	**Immunohistochemical marker**
Carcinoma	Cytokeratin, EMA
Lymphoma	CLA, EMA
Sarcoma	Vimentin, desmin, factor VIII antigen
Melanoma	S-100, HMB-45, vimentin, NSE
Neuroendocrine	Chromogranin, synaptophysin, cytokeratin, EMA, NSE
Germ cell tumour	Cytokeratin, HCG, AFP, EMA
Prostate cancer	Cytokeratin, PSA, EMA
Breast cancer	Cytokeratin, ER, PR, EMA
Thyroid cancer	Thyroglobulin, cytokeratin, EMA, calcitonin
CLA, common leucocyte antigen; EMA, epithelial membrane antigen; NSE, neuron specific enolase.	

Table 2 **Differential cytokeratin (CK) staining**		
	CK20 positive	**CK20 negative**
CK7 positive	Transitional cell carcinoma	Breast cancer
	Pancreatic carcinoma	Non-small cell lung cancer
	Ovarian mucinous adenocarcinoma	Ovarian serous carcinoma
	Merkel cell carcinoma	Mesothelioma
		Endometrial cancer
		Pancreatic cancer
CK7 negative	Colorectal cancer	Hepatocellular
		Renal cell cancer
		Prostate cancer
		SCC
		Neuroendocrine carcinoma

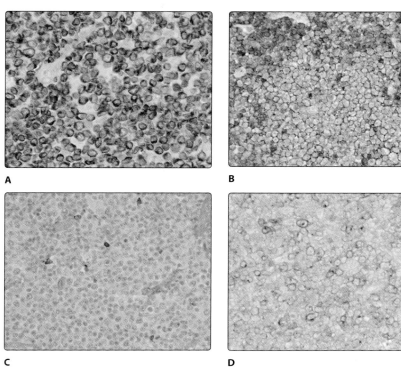

A   **B**

C   **D**

Fig. 1 **Immunohistochemical stains** – upper level CD3 and CD4, lower level CD8, CD25. Imaging shows a CD3/CD4/CD25 positive malignancy which is also CD8 negative.

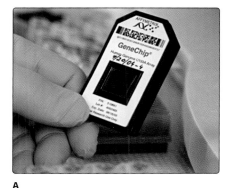

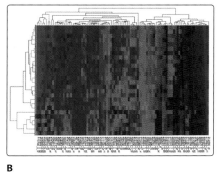

A   **B**

Fig. 2 **DNA microarray** may be assessed using chip technology (figure A). It is a collection of microscopic DNA spots attached to a solid surface, such as for the purpose of monitoring expression levels for thousands of genes simultaneously. Green or blue (in this figure blue) represents up-regulation, while red indicates down-regulation.

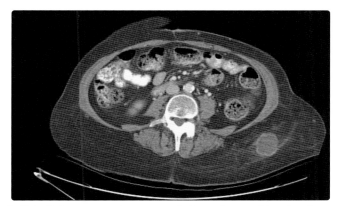

Fig. 3 **A soft clinically innocuous subcutaneous lesion on immunohistochemistry** was consistent with melanoma metastases, although no primary was identified.

crucial to identify those treatment-responsive presentations of unknown primary with the greatest potential for long-term survival.

Management

The majority of patients have disseminated disease; options depend on the particular clinical scenario. It appears there are certain subsets of CUP that may be more responsive to intervention.

- Poorly differentiated midline tumours may respond to platinum chemotherapy in 50% of cases, with 10–15% having long-term durable responses. HCG and AFP should be assessed and followed if increased.
- A female patient with axillary lymph node involvement with adenocarcinoma should be considered as having breast cancer, with appropriate combination therapy – axillary resection, radiation, chemotherapy or hormonal therapy; 5- and 10-year overall survival rates of 75% and 60%, respectively, have been documented.
- Squamous carcinoma of cervical lymph nodes is treated as head and neck cancer.
- Peritoneal carcinomatosis in women should be treated as ovarian cancer.
- Men with osteoblastic metastases and elevated PSA levels should be treated as prostate cancer.

Carcinoma of unknown primary

- Cancer of unknown primary occurs in 3–5% of patients with metastatic disease.
- Careful attention to detail is important.
- Immunohistochemistry, electron microscopy, microarray and laboratory findings may be of help.
- Investigations are targeted to identify treatable options.
- Median survival is 3–4 months.

Neutropenic sepsis

This constitutes one of the most common oncological emergencies encountered by oncology staff. Prior to the availability of broad spectrum antibiotics and growth factors, infections were responsible for 75% of chemotherapy-related mortality.

Definition of neutropenic fever

Neutropenic fever is defined as a temperature of >38.5°C on one occasion or a temperature of 38.0°C on two occasions over an hour in a patient with an absolute neutrophil count (ANC) less than 500 cells/µL.

The presence of fever and neutropenia does not imply sepsis:

- only 10–20% will have microbiologically documented infection
- 20–30% may have clinically documented infections such as cellulitis, pneumonia, typhlitis
- 50–70% will have no clinical or microbiological evidence of infection.

Risk factors for infection

The absolute ANC nadir, duration and rate of decline all impact on the absolute infection risk and associated morbidity. Other predisposing factors are:

- impaired cell-mediated and humoral immunity related to certain underlying disease states – lymphoma, leukaemia and myeloma and therapies
- increased risk of encapsulated bacterial infections in splenectomised patients
- mucositis, which may occur as a toxicity of chemotherapy or radiation therapy, increasing the risk of seeding of the bloodstream by gastrointestinal pathogens
- implanted devices (vascular access devices or stents); these may become colonised and lead to local infection
- disease-causing obstruction such as lung mass, which may facilitate local infection causing a post-obstructive pneumonia.

Clinical presentation

Neutropenic patients may develop sepsis in the absence of a fever, particularly with the concurrent administration of steroids or in the elderly. The absence of neutrophils often prevents the development of overt local signs or symptoms; therefore succinct history and thorough physical examination are essential.

Physical examination includes inspection of skin, sinuses, fundi, oropharynx, lung, abdomen, perineum, mucous membranes and any vascular access devices. Internal examinations (vaginal, rectal) or instrumentation (urinary catheter) are relatively contraindicated due to the risk of introducing infection.

As the ANC recovers, signs and symptoms of infection usually become evident. Repeat examinations and assessments should be performed daily.

Investigations

Every patient should have complete blood count with differential, hepatic and renal function, urinalysis, chest X-ray and cultures – blood, urine, sputum and throat.

Standard practice for blood cultures:

- Adequate volume of blood (at least 10 mL) is required for microbiological assessment.
- Aerobic and anaerobic blood culture bottles should be obtained.
- A minimum of two sets of cultures should be obtained.
- In the case of a vascular access device with multiple lumens, all lumens should be cultured.
- Cultures should be repeated at regular intervals for persistent fevers or chills.

In patients with localising signs or symptoms, more specific investigations may be warranted:

- With upper respiratory tract symptoms, a nasopharyngeal wash for respiratory syncytial virus, adenovirus, cytomegalovirus (CMV), influenza A and B and parainfluenza virus 1, 2 and 3 should be completed (Fig. 1).
- With diarrhoea, stool for ova, cysts, parasites and *Clostridium difficile* toxin should be sent.

Appropriate imaging should be performed to visualise sinuses, chest, abdomen or pelvis. Bronchoscopy should be considered in a patient with

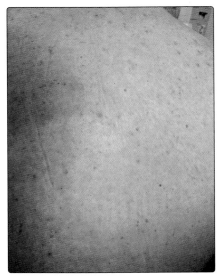

Fig. 1 **Viral exanthema** – a non-specific erythematous maculopapular rash in a patient with prolonged profound neutropenia and serum CMV PCR (polymerase chain reaction) positive.

Box 1 Antibiotic choice in special clinical circumstances

Penicillin allergic patients
(a) Aztreonam and vancomycin
Abdominal pain (typhlitis)
(a) Imipenem or
(b) Meropenem or
(c) Cephalosporin and metronidazole
Pulmonary infiltrate in febrile neutropenia
(a) Imipenem or
(b) Meropenem or } and fluoroquinolone
(c) Cephalosporin

---

pulmonary lesions failing to improve on empiric antibiotics.

Management

Immediate evaluation of patients is mandatory. Initial coverage is aimed at bacterial infections. There are certain antibiotic choices in special clinical circumstances (Box 1). However, in general, no specific antibiotic regimen has been shown to be superior, but the approach to each patient requires individualisation, taking account of certain features.

- *In a clinically stable patient – uncomplicated fever and neutropenia.* Intravenous monotherapy with an anti-pseudomonal β-lactam is recommended. Combination of a β-lactam and aminoglycoside has been associated with more toxicity without superior outcome. It is important to be familiar with the pattern of antibiotic resistance in the particular institution.

- *When is vancomycin required?*
  There are certain indications for vancomycin use – severe sepsis or shock, clinically apparent catheter-related infection, known colonisation with methicillin-resistant *Staphylococcus aureus* (MRSA) or severe mucositis.
- *If sepsis or shock is present.*
  In the setting of severe sepsis, broad spectrum coverage for Gram-negative bacilli and viridans group streptococci should be initiated; dual therapy with either β-lactam and aminoglycoside or β-lactam and fluoroquinolone maximises antimicrobial coverage. Vancomycin is also added empirically in this situation.
- *What to do with persistent fever in a stable patient.*
  If the fever resolves then antibiotics are continued until the ANC is ≥500/mm³. For clinical or microbiological proven infection, antibiotics are continued for the appropriate standard length of time.
  If fever persists but the patient remains neutropenic and clinically stable, the initial antibiotic regimen should continue while performing daily physical examinations and cultures. Antifungal therapy should be added in the face of persistent fevers and neutropenia for a period greater than 4 days.
- *What if the fevers continue but the patient's condition deteriorates?*
  Change the antimicrobials and investigate exhaustively for possible fungal infection.

Fungal infections

Invasive fungal infections are uncommon early in the course of neutropenia, but the risk increases with duration and degree of neutropenia. Certain haematological malignancies are also associated with immunocompromise, thus increasing the risk of fungal infections (Fig. 2). Candida infection tends to appear earlier than mould infection. Fungal infections can be difficult to diagnose and are associated with high mortality; therefore the addition of antifungal therapy in neutropenic fever after a

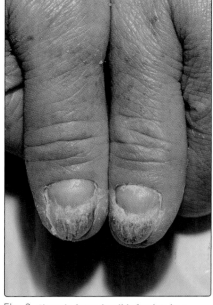

Fig. 2 **Chronic fungal nail infection in a patient with lymphoma.**

specified time period has become standard. Diagnosis of antifungal pulmonary infection requires a CT scan of the chest and serum galactomannan antigen as a minimum. The choice of the antifungal agent should be based on the clinical picture.
Indications for antifungals are:

- persistent fever after 4–7 days of antibacterial agents
- new fever after defervescence
- new pulmonary infiltrates while on broad spectrum antibiotics
- isolation of yeast from a sterile site or mould from any site.

Catheter-related infections

Vascular access devices are required in many patients to facilitate administration of chemotherapy; however, these devices remain an important source of sepsis. The most common organisms causing catheter-related infections are documented in Table 1. A variety of clinical situations may occur:

- catheter colonisation – significant growth of an organism from the culture of the catheter tip or hub
- exit site infection – erythema, induration and tenderness within 2 cm of the catheter exit site with or without bloodstream infection
- tunnel infection – erythema, induration and tenderness within 12 cm from the catheter exit site along the subcutaneous tract of the tunnelled device with or without bloodstream infection

- pocket infection – infected fluid in the subcutaneous pocket of a totally implanted intravascular device with or without bloodstream infection
- catheter-related bloodstream infection – bacteraemia or fungaemia in a patient with an intravascular device and one positive result from culture of blood samples from the periphery.

Granulocyte colony-stimulating factors

Granulocyte colony-stimulating factors (G-CSFs) should only be considered in critically ill patients or those whose bone marrow recovery is expected to be prolonged. Indications for primary prophylaxis are outlined in Box 2.

Table 1 **Organisms causing catheter-related infections**

Organism	Frequency
Coagulase-negative staphylococci	37%
Enterococci	14%
S. aureus	12%
Gram-negative bacilli	14%
Candida infection	8%

> ### Box 2 Indications for G-CSF primary prophylaxis
>
> - If probability of febrile neutropenia >40%
> - If dose reduction is considered detrimental
> - Elderly frail patients
> - Chemotherapy with active infection
> - Reduced marrow reserve
> - HIV

> **Neutropenic sepsis**
>
> - This is a medical oncology emergency.
> - It is a rise in temperature of >38.5°C once or 38.0°C on two occasions in a patient with an ANC less than 500 cells/μL.
> - Failure to start antibiotics in the first 24 hours may result in mortality rates of 80%. Empiric antibiotics are imperative.
> - It requires careful history and examination.
> - Regular reassessment is necessary to detect clinical changes.
> - An organism will be identified in only 10–20% of cases.

Spinal cord compression

Spinal cord compression is a potentially devastating event that may result in severe neurological impairment. The most important intervention is speedy diagnosis and prompt treatment. Neurological outcome is dependent on the speed of intervention and the neurological function at the time of treatment.

Anatomy

The spinal cord, enclosed within the thecal sac, is protected by the bones of the vertebral column. Normally, the thecal sac is surrounded by the epidural space. Compression is a mechanical phenomenon most commonly caused by tumour invading the epidural space and growing within the unyielding bony confines of the spinal canal, as illustrated in Fig. 1. Compression of the epidural venous plexus produces vasogenic oedema within the cord and ultimately leads to ischaemia and cell death, at which time the neurological damage is irreversible. Intramedullary or leptomeningeal tumours are much rarer causes of compression.

In the adult, the spinal cord ends at the level of L1. The spinal nerves below this level comprise the cauda equina, which is subject to compression by the same mechanisms as the spinal cord.

Aetiology

Vertebral bone metastases associated with breast, prostate and lung cancer account for the majority of cases. Lymphoma, multiple myeloma, renal cell carcinoma and sarcoma are also associated with cord compression. Approximately 20% of patients presenting with spinal cord compression have no known history of malignant disease and require investigation to establish the site of the primary cancer. Patients with cancer may also present with benign causes of spinal cord compression including epidural abscess and vertebral disc prolapse.

Symptoms and signs

Unfortunately delay in diagnosis is the norm, even in patients with a known history of malignancy who are therefore at high risk for spinal cord compression. Increased awareness among patients and medical staff regarding the importance of back pain and defined investigative procedures for the patient with back pain in combination with neurological symptoms may help to promote earlier intervention.

Back pain is the commonest symptom, occurring in almost all patients before neurological symptoms. Loss of sensation and muscle weakness below the level of the lesion are characteristic neurological signs. Careful examination may reveal a sensory level. Although this level approximates the actual level of compression, it is not an accurate indicator and should not be used to guide treatment. Muscle weakness follows a lower motor neuron pattern and is usually progressive and symmetrical. Bladder and bowel dysfunction may manifest as urinary retention and constipation.

Diagnosis

Magnetic resonance imaging of the entire spine is the investigation of choice. Ideally the entire spine should be visualised as lesions occur at more than one level in approximately 25% of cases. MRI produces high resolution images of the thecal sac compression, as illustrated in Fig. 2, as well as visualising the paraspinal tissues. CT myelography involves injection of contrast media into the spinal canal via lumbar puncture and is useful in patients with a contraindication to MRI, for example those with a mechanical heart valve.

A histological diagnosis must be established for those presenting with spinal cord compression as the first manifestation of malignant disease. This can be done by image-guided needle biopsy of the vertebral lesion. Investigations aimed at defining the primary site can be conducted as indicated after treatment for spinal cord compression has been initiated.

Management

Many patients with spinal cord compression have metastatic disease associated with a poor prognosis. Delay in diagnosis means that many patients are unable to walk at the time of presentation and are unlikely to regain full neurological function. In this scenario, treatment options should be tailored to individual cases.

Corticosteroids, surgery, radiotherapy and systemic treatment may all play a role in management. Patients with a poor performance status are usually treated with corticosteroids and

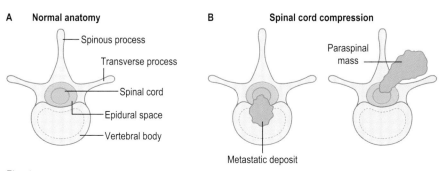

A **Normal anatomy**
- Spinous process
- Transverse process
- Spinal cord
- Epidural space
- Vertebral body

B **Spinal cord compression**
- Metastatic deposit
- Paraspinal mass

Fig. 1 **Mechanism of spinal cord compression.**

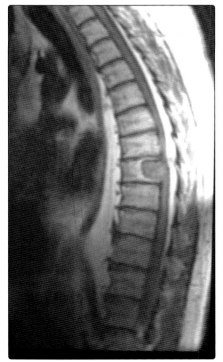

Fig. 2 **Spinal cord compression on MRI.**

radiotherapy. Carefully selected patients may benefit from neurosurgery, which can be followed by radiotherapy. Adequate analgesia should be provided as almost all patients present with pain.

Steroids

Intravenous dexamethasone is a standard component in the treatment of spinal cord compression. It is likely that dexamethasone works by reducing vasogenic oedema, thus relieving compression to some degree. Doses as high as 100 mg per day have been used and although efficacious, are associated with severe side effects; 16 mg per day in divided doses is a more typical regimen. Consideration can be given to tapering the dexamethasone dose when the patient has commenced definitive treatment and is neurologically stable.

Radiotherapy

The radiation field is usually 8 cm wide and includes the level of obstruction with one or two vertebrae above and below the lesion. Various fractionation regimens have been used ranging from 40 Gy in 20 fractions to hypofractionated regimens such as 30 Gy in 10 fractions or 20 Gy in 5 fractions. Patients with poor performance status may be treated with a single fraction. There are no randomised trials identifying the optimal regimen. Treatment regimen is often chosen based on individual patient characteristics such as likelihood of response, general condition and prognosis.

Surgery

Radical surgery is beneficial in a selected group of patients who have good performance status, short duration of paraparesis and a reasonable life expectancy. It is also useful in specific situations as described in Box 1. Procedures performed include anterior or posterior decompression and spinal stabilisation by bone graft or insertion of synthetic material.

Systemic therapy

Appropriate systemic treatment should be initiated in tandem with local treatment. There is no evidence that local therapy can be omitted even for chemosensitive tumours such as lymphoma. Chemotherapy in conjunction with steroids may be used in patients not considered suitable for radiotherapy or surgery.

Prognosis

Very few patients with paraplegia regain the ability to walk after treatment, underlining the importance of diagnosis prior to the onset of severe neurological impairment. The median survival from time of diagnosis is 3 to 6 months.

Box 1 Specific indications for surgical decompression

- No histological diagnosis
- Spinal instability
- Dislodged bone fragments causing compression
- Previous radiotherapy such that further radiotherapy cannot be given
- Tumour resistant to radiotherapy and chemotherapy
- Neurological deterioration while patient on radiotherapy

Spinal cord compression

- Spinal cord compression is an emergency.
- Early diagnosis and rapid treatment are of paramount importance.
- The most common malignant causes are breast, lung and prostate cancer.
- Most patients are treated with a combination of radiotherapy and high dose intravenous dexamethasone.
- Surgery is performed in selected cases.
- Functional outcome is dependent on the neurological state at the time of treatment.

Superior vena cava obstruction

Superior vena cava obstruction (SVCO) usually presents with gradual onset of symptoms in a patient with stable vital signs at the time of presentation. This allows time for investigation, diagnosis and appropriate treatment of the underlying cause of the obstruction. The outcome of treatment most often depends on the diagnosis and the stage of the underlying disease, not on the immediate institution of treatment. Historically, urgent radiotherapy was often given prior to full work-up – this approach no longer represents best practice.

A minority of cases present with acute SVCO and associated compression of the trachea resulting in stridor and respiratory compromise. These cases are true emergencies and will require urgent treatment to relieve the obstruction.

Aetiology

Obstruction of the superior vena cava can be caused by extrinsic compression of the vessel, most commonly caused by malignancy, or blockage within the vessel lumen as in the case of thrombosis. Over 80% of cases are caused by an underlying malignancy with infection and thrombosis accounting for most of the remaining cases. SVCO may be the first manifestation of malignancy. Causative conditions are listed in Box 1.

History and examination

The speed of progression of symptoms is dependent on the rate of obstruction and the development of collateral vessels to circumvent the obstruction. Sudden obstruction precludes the development of collateral vessels and results in rapid onset of symptoms. In most cases, symptoms appear over a period of days or weeks.

Symptoms include shortness of breath, headache and swelling of the face and neck. Dizziness and swelling of the arm or breast may also occur. On examination distended veins may be apparent on the neck and chest wall. Raised jugular venous pressure may be present. Systematic examination may reveal enlarged supraclavicular or axillary lymph nodes, which will make a convenient biopsy target in cases with no previous history of malignancy. Pemberton's sign may be positive – shortness of breath, stridor or facial plethora occurring on raising the arms above the head and keeping them there for one minute.

Investigation and diagnosis

The aim of investigation is two-fold: to confirm the diagnosis of SVCO and to identify the underlying cause.

Radiology

- Chest X-ray – the majority of patients with underlying malignancy will have abnormal findings such as a lung mass, widened mediastinum or pleural effusion.
- CT scan of the chest – appearances on CT scan will usually suggest an underlying diagnosis. CT is also used as a staging investigation for lung cancer and lymphoma.
- Venography – injection and imaging of contrast in the veins of the upper limbs provides detailed information regarding the level and extent of obstruction and the pattern of collateral blood flow. This procedure is diagnostic in the case of thrombosis and may be therapeutic if a stent is inserted to relieve the obstruction.

Histological diagnosis

Patients with radiological findings suggestive of malignancy require a biopsy to establish a histological diagnosis prior to treatment. The best approach depends on the individual situation. Common sampling procedures include the following:

- sputum or pleural fluid cytology
- bronchoscopy or CT-guided transthoracic biopsy for sampling a lung lesion
- mediastinoscopy for a mediastinal mass.

Management

Emergency

SVCO may be accompanied by obstruction of the trachea. Patients who present with stridor require urgent intervention to prevent progression to cardiorespiratory arrest. Insertion of a stent in the trachea and/or the SVC provides rapid relief.

Malignant obstruction

Dexamethasone reduces oedema and provides symptomatic relief in patients with malignant obstruction. Doses in the range 12–16 mg daily are commonly given. The indications for further treatment will depend on the nature of the underlying malignancy. Treatment options may be limited by previous treatment in the case of progressive or recurrent disease.

There is evidence that mechanical relief of the obstruction by insertion of a stent provides more rapid relief in a higher proportion of patients than treatment with either chemotherapy or radiotherapy. Intraluminal stenting is performed in the radiology department under fluoroscopic guidance, a service which may not always be available. This procedure may be particularly useful in certain situations, as listed in Box 2. Although stenting may provide relief of symptoms it does not treat the underlying malignancy.

Box 1 Causes of SVCO

Primary malignant disease:
- Lung cancer – small cell lung cancer is more likely to cause SVCO than is non-small cell lung cancer
- Lymphoma
- Thymoma
- Germ cell tumours arising in the mediastinum

Secondary malignant disease:
- Mediastinal lymph node metastases due to solid tumours, e.g. breast cancer, lung cancer

Non-malignant causes:
- Infection
- Thrombosis
- Fibrosis after thoracic radiation

Box 2 Specific indications for stenting

- Patient unlikely to tolerate radiotherapy and/or chemotherapy
- Tumour not responsive to chemotherapy or radiotherapy
- Tumour within a previously irradiated area, precluding further radiotherapy
- Patient refusing chemotherapy and radiotherapy

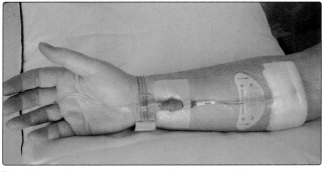

Fig. 1 **Indwelling central venous catheter inserted through a peripheral vein.**

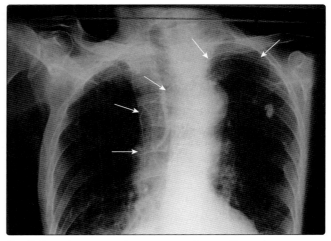

Fig. 2 **Central venous catheter seen on chest radiograph.**

The definitive treatment of underlying malignancy is dealt with in the relevant chapters. Malignancies which are sensitive to chemotherapy may respond quite rapidly, producing relief of symptoms. Lymphoma, small cell lung cancer and primary mediastinal germ cell tumours may be treated in the first instance with chemotherapy with or without radiotherapy.

Patients with a poor performance status and a poor prognosis based on stage of disease are treated with palliative intent. Radiotherapy is often delivered in this setting as it is well tolerated and produces useful palliation of symptoms. A short hypofractionated course of treatment is commonly prescribed, such as 20 Gy given in five fractions over 5 days.

Thrombosis

Thrombosis is a well-recognised complication of indwelling central venous catheters. The clot may occur in the upper extremity veins or the SVC depending on the placement of the catheter. Various designs of catheter are in current clinical use, one of which is illustrated in Fig. 1. Catheter placement is checked on chest radiograph (Fig. 2).

Thrombolytic therapy should be administered in the form of heparin followed by oral anticoagulation with warfarin. This may be given while the catheter remains in place to complete chemotherapy if required. Alternatively, the catheter can be removed, followed by short-term anticoagulation. Standard contraindications to anticoagulation apply. In addition, the following cases are of particular concern in the oncology setting:

- primary or secondary intracranial malignancy
- a primary tumour which may bleed profusely
- impaired liver function
- drug interactions, e.g. warfarin and chemotherapeutic agents or antibiotics.

Superior vena cava obstruction

- Malignancy is the most common cause of SVCO.
- SVCO may be the first presentation of malignancy.
- The chest radiograph is usually abnormal.
- Most cases do not require emergency treatment.
- Definitive diagnosis prior to treatment is the correct management approach in clinically stable patients.

Metabolic emergencies

There are a number of different metabolic emergencies in medical oncology; they arise as a result of the cancer, as well as treatment. This chapter will discuss the more important emergencies such as hypercalcaemia and tumour lysis syndrome.

Hypercalcaemia

Hypercalcaemia may occur in 10–20% of cancer patients and treatment can be associated with significant improvement in quality of life and reduced morbidity. The most common malignancies associated with hypercalcaemia include breast and lung cancer, kidney cancer, myeloma, lymphoma, and head and neck cancers. A rare malignant cause of hypercalcaemia is parathyroid cancer.

Aetiology

There are many causes of hypercalcaemia.

- 80% of patients with hypercalcaemia have bone metastases; the extent of disease does not correlate with calcium levels. Direct bone destruction mobilises calcium but indirect destruction occurs as a result of osteoclast-activating factors.
  - Parathyroid hormone (PTH)-related peptide secreted into the circulation by lung and breast cancer, lymphoma, and squamous cell carcinomas of the head and neck. It not only causes bone resorption but also increases renal calcium reabsorption.
  - Prostaglandins produced by patients with lung, kidney and ovarian cancer.
  - Transforming growth factor (TGF) and IL-6 found commonly in myeloma.

A large number of patients have lytic bone lesions; however, only a fraction of these develop hypercalcaemia, thus other factors interplay (Fig. 1).

- Decreased calcium excretion may occur as a result of renal disease or the effects of the circulating factors.
- There may be increased production of calcitriol by cancer cells, particularly lymphoma.

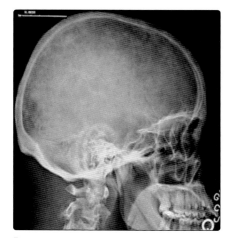

Fig. 1 **Lytic metastatic bone disease causing hypercalcaemia.**

Clinical presentation

The severity of the symptoms depends on both the absolute calcium value and the rate of increase. Some patients with bone metastases from breast cancer develop hypercalcaemia so insidiously that they tolerate very high values.

The classic symptoms include:

- nausea and vomiting
- anorexia
- constipation
- dehydration
- polyuria and polydipsia
- muscle weakness
- chemical conjunctivitis (Fig. 2)
- confusion
- coma.

Management

Patients with severe hypercalcaemia require emergent therapy. Initial management consists of aggressive hydration with infusion of 4–6 litres in the first 24 hours. Loop diuretics are proposed as a calcium-lowering agent. However, these should not be added until the patient is volume replete.

Specific hypocalcaemic agents should be administered:

- *Bisphosphonates* are analogues of pyrophosphate that bind to bone hydroxyapatite; the compounds are taken up by the osteoclast and inhibit its action, preventing bone resorption. Many agents are available clinically but for all, the beneficial effects are not seen for 3–4 days, while the effect may last for 7–30 days. Hypocalcaemia,

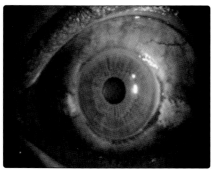

Fig. 2 **Hypercalcaemia-induced conjunctivitis.**

hypomagnesaemia and hypophosphataemia is seen in >10% of patients.

- *Calcitonin* is capable of rapidly reducing calcium levels within 24 hours of therapy although its effects are often short lived; it should be used in conjunction with longer acting agents such as bisphosphonates. Usual dose is 4 IU/kg intramuscularly or subcutaneously every 12 hours but tachyphylaxis often develops with prolonged therapy.
- *Gallium nitrate* prevents bone resorption; dosing requires intravenous infusion for 5 consecutive days and calcium values may normalise for 10–14 days.
- *Steroids* are of benefit in patients with steroid-responsive cancers such as myeloma and lymphoma by blocking bone resorption.
- *Mithramycin* was used more frequently prior to the introduction of bisphosphonates; thrombocytopenia and nephrotoxicity limit its use.

Treatment of the underlying disease with anticancer therapy is the most beneficial step in managing hypercalcaemia in the long term.

Tumour lysis syndrome

Tumour lysis syndrome (TLS) is a medical oncology emergency where cell lysis occurs, resulting in the massive release of intracellular contents into the systemic circulation. It may occur spontaneously in cancers with high proliferative rates, as a response to highly effective therapy.

It is a constellation of metabolic abnormalities which may result in renal failure, cardiac arrhythmias, seizure or death:

- hyperuricaemia
- hyperkalaemia
- hypocalcaemia
- hyperphosphataemia.

Certain cancers have a greater predisposition such as lymphomas, leukaemias, small cell lung cancer and multiple myeloma. Certain features place a patient at greater risk (Box 1).

Box 1 Risk factors for TLS

- Lymphoproliferative malignancies
- Bulky disease
- Elevated lactate dehydrogenase
- Elevated white cell count
- Renal impairment
- Elevated uric acid
- Dehydration

Evaluation

Serial measurement of electrolytes, BUN (blood, urea, nitrogen), creatinine, calcium, phosphorus and uric acid must be obtained. In high-risk cases these levels are monitored every 6 hours. The lethal complication is arrhythmias secondary to hyperkalaemia and hypocalcaemia.

Management

Recognising high-risk patients and initiating prophylactic measures to prevent TLS is essential. If possible, for the 48 hours prior to therapy patients should receive:

- allopurinol – decreases uric acid production by competitively inhibiting xanthine oxidase
- vigorous hydration to ensure high urine volumes
- urinary alkalinisation with sodium bicarbonate to maintain a pH >7.

Drugs that interfere with tubular reabsorption of uric acid (aspirin, radiographic contrast and thiazides) should be avoided. If oliguria develops, a renal ultrasound should be performed to rule out ureteral obstruction. Urinary catheterisation may be needed to accurately monitor urine output.

Hyperkalaemia may require treatment with calcium gluconate, dextrose and insulin or calcium resonium. If acute renal failure ensues, dialysis should be commenced. Hyperphosphataemia is treated with a phosphate binder, while hypocalcaemia only requires intervention if the patient is symptomatic.

Metabolic emergencies

- Hypercalcaemia results in significant morbidity and mortality.
- Effective management can improve quality of life significantly.
- Tumour lysis syndrome is a preventable emergency in many cases.

Pain management

Fear of pain, particularly towards the end of life, is often a major worry for cancer patients and their carers. The majority of patients with cancer will experience pain during the course of their illness, particularly if they develop metastatic disease. Successful relief of pain is possible for most patients and should be the aim of treatment.

Types of cancer pain

- Somatic pain – this results from direct injury to tissues with pain well localised to the site of the injury often associated with tenderness. Bone metastases are a common example.
- Visceral pain – pain emanating from an organ is classically dull and colicky in nature and is less well localised. Associated symptoms such as nausea and sweating may occur. It is often referred to a cutaneous area sharing innervation with the organ. The classic example of this is pain due to diaphragmatic irritation referred to the point of the shoulder. Pain due to pancreatic cancer or small bowel obstruction is visceral in nature.
- Neuropathic pain – this may result from direct infiltration or compression of nerves, resulting in shooting, burning pain which may be associated with tingling, numbness and altered sensation in the area supplied by the nerve. Examples include nerve root compression or brachial plexopathy.

Pain assessment

Accurate and repeated assessment of pain is vital to successful relief of symptoms. History and examination should help uncover the likely cause. Key questions which should be asked are listed in Box 1. Many cancer patients have multiple pain symptoms each of which should be explored. Once appropriate treatment has been instituted, symptoms should be reassessed to determine response.

In the clinic the patient can be asked to rate their pain on a categorical scale (none, mild, moderate or severe) or to indicate on a visual scale (Fig. 1) how they rate their pain.

Management

A realistic plan tailored to the individual patient should be defined

Box 1 History taking – key questions

- Where is the pain?
- Does it radiate to any other site?
- When did the pain start?
- Is the pain improving or worsening?
- Describe the character of the pain.
- Does anything make the pain better or worse?
  Incident pain is due to a clear precipitating cause.
  Breakthrough pain is not associated with an identifiable cause.
- Are there any associated symptoms?
- What analgesics have been used and did they help?
- Did previous analgesics cause side effects?
- What impact is the pain having on daily activities?

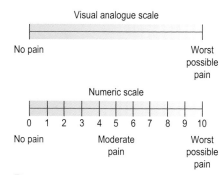

Fig. 1 **Visual assessment of pain severity.**

at the outset. Patients benefit from a multidisciplinary approach drawing on palliative care, oncology, surgery and anaesthetic skills as well as psychologists, dieticians, physiotherapists and occupational therapists. Treatment modalities include the following:

- anticancer therapy
- analgesics
- adjuvant treatments
- surgery
- nerve blocks
- non-pharmacological interventions.

Anticancer therapy

Chemotherapy

Second and third line chemotherapy regimens are associated with reducing rates of response in patients with

progressive disease after first line therapy. However, in the setting of widely disseminated metastatic disease with severe symptoms, systemic therapy may be indicated in those cancers which are sensitive, e.g. haematological malignancies.

Hormone therapy

Prostate cancer and breast cancer are common causes of diffuse bone metastases. Both are sensitive to hormonal therapy. Previously untreated advanced prostate cancer frequently shows excellent response to therapy with gonadotrophin releasing hormone agonists. Responses may also be seen with second line hormonal therapy in both breast and prostate cancer.

Radiotherapy

Pain due to localised tumour infiltration and pressure can be treated very effectively by radiotherapy. It is one of the single most effective treatments for bone metastases but is also useful in the treatment of pain due to recurrent or progressive tumour masses (e.g. pelvic disease), primary or metastatic brain lesions and pathological fractures (in conjunction with surgery). External beam radiotherapy is most commonly used. Radioisotopes such as strontium and samarium may be used in the treatment of diffuse bone metastases.

Analgesics

WHO analgesic ladder

The analgesic ladder (Fig. 2) was designed as a tool to guide the administration of analgesics with a view to optimal pain relief. Medication should be given regularly, not just when pain is severe and should be given by mouth if possible. Side effects should be sought and treated proactively so that the dose can be titrated upwards while minimising adverse effects. Medication should be provided for breakthrough pain. The patient should be frequently reassessed and adjuvant treatment given as appropriate. While it is frequently reasonable to proceed through steps 1 to 3, prescribing strong opioids such as morphine may be necessary in the first instance for patients with severe pain at first presentation.

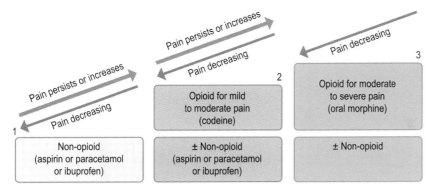

Fig. 2 **WHO analgesic ladder.**

Within Fig. 2:
- Pain persists or increases
- Pain decreasing
- 1
- Non-opioid (aspirin or paracetamol or ibuprofen)
- Pain persists or increases
- Pain decreasing
- 2
- Opioid for mild to moderate pain (codeine)
- ± Non-opioid (aspirin or paracetamol or ibuprofen)
- Pain decreasing
- 3
- Opioid for moderate to severe pain (oral morphine)
- ± Non-opioid

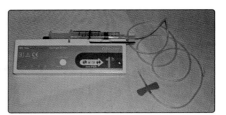

Fig. 3 **Syringe driver.**

Prescription of opioids

A patient who has not taken opioids before (referred to as opioid naïve) is usually prescribed 5–10 mg of rapid-acting morphine formulation to be taken by mouth every 4 hours. This dose is titrated upwards to achieve control of symptoms. The total daily dose can then be given as a sustained release preparation, i.e. a twice daily dose of 12-hourly morphine. Rapid-acting morphine should always be available to the patient for treatment of breakthrough pain whenever it is required. The sustained release dose can be adjusted according to the demand for additional breakthrough doses.

Parenteral administration can be considered in patients unable to take morphine orally. For ongoing pain relief, the use of a syringe driver (Fig. 3) is the preferred method of drug delivery. Parenteral administration of morphine increases its bioavailability and the dose should be adjusted accordingly. As a rule of thumb, the oral dose should be halved when switching to the parenteral route. Fentanyl is marketed as a transdermal patch, which may be ideal for patients on a stable dose of morphine. Hydromorphone, oxycodone and fentanyl are all more potent than morphine to varying degrees, which must be carefully accounted for when prescribing or when switching formulations.

Side effects of opioids

In the palliative care setting, nausea, vomiting and constipation are the most commonly encountered side effects. Constipation is best prevented by prophylactic administration of a laxative with opioids, with regular review of bowel habit. Confusion, tremors, hallucinations and respiratory depression may occur with toxic doses. Reduction of the dose or discontinuation of morphine will relieve symptoms of toxicity. This should be done in concert with additional pain control measures to prevent pain symptoms recurring. Naloxone, an antidote to opioids, may be prescribed in an emergency situation.

Adjuvant therapies

Adjuvant drugs should be considered at all stages of the analgesic ladder. They may have a direct analgesic effect or may relieve other symptoms such as nausea and anxiety which adversely affect the patient's perception of pain.

- Benzodiazepines are useful in the treatment of anxiety, fear and insomnia in the cancer patient. Midazolam may be used in syringe drivers for anxiety associated with terminal disease.
- Chlorpromazine and haloperidol may be indicated for antiemetic and sedative effects.
- Antidepressants – amitriptyline is indicated in the treatment of neuropathic pain.
- Anticonvulsants are useful in the treatment of post-herpetic neuralgia, postoperative pain and neuropathic pain characterised by sharp, stabbing pain and tingling. Older agents include carbamazepine, phenytoin and sodium valproate. Gabapentin, a newer agent, is now commonly used.
- Corticosteroids are frequently used for their anti-inflammatory effects, which may reduce swelling and pressure symptoms.
- Bisphosphonates, which are available in intravenous and oral preparations, are proven to reduce bone pain and the incidence of vertebral fracture in patients with bone metastases.

Surgery

Pathological fractures may require surgical fixation. Occasionally a large bone lesion with a high risk of fracture will be stabilised as a preventive measure. Other indications for surgical intervention include bypass procedures to relieve obstructive symptoms in the bowel, spinal stabilisation, insertion of stents, insertion of shunts to relieve obstructive hydrocephalus and rarely ablative procedures for the patient who has intractable pain in spite of medical management.

Nerve blocks

Pain localised to one nerve or nerve plexus can be relieved by nerve block – injection of local anaesthetic in the vicinity of the nerve. The effect of the anaesthetic wears off in a matter of hours. Long-term relief can be achieved by insertion of a catheter or injection of an agent such as phenol which damages the nerve. The latter method produces sensory and motor loss within the distribution of the nerve. Visceral pain responds well to such interventions, e.g. coeliac plexus block for pancreatic cancer pain.

Non-pharmacological methods

Transcutaneous electrical nerve stimulation (TENS) machines may provide substantial relief from neuropathic pain. Acupuncture often provides temporary relief for interested patients. Physiotherapy, application of cold/heat and psychological methods may be helpful.

Pain management

- Most cancer patients experience pain during the course of their illness.
- Analgesics should be introduced according to the analgesic ladder.
- The goal of treatment should be optimal pain relief with minimal side effects.
- A multidisciplinary approach should be adopted.

Specific metastatic conditions

This chapter reviews treatment options for metastatic disease to specific organs. Appropriate cytotoxic treatment for the underlying malignancy should be considered for all of these conditions and is dealt with in the relevant chapters throughout the book. These comments apply to metastatic disease in general.

Bone metastases

Bone metastases are a common manifestation of advanced disease in breast, prostate and lung cancer. Patients who have bone metastases but no visceral metastases may live for long periods of time, during which their quality of life may be significantly impaired by pain, immobility and potential complications such as spinal cord compression, pathological fracture and hypercalcaemia. Optimal management of bone metastases improves quality of life and reduces the incidence of events such as fracture.

The medical oncologist, palliative care team, radiation oncologist, surgeon, physiotherapist and occupational therapist among others all have a role to play. Any patient with a known history of malignancy, presenting with pain suggestive of bone metastases, should have plain radiographs and a bone scan performed. A sudden increase in pain may indicate pathological fracture which can occur in the absence of trauma. The management of pain and specific therapy for the underlying malignancy are outlined in the relevant chapters. Other aspects of treatment will be dealt with here.

Metastatic lesions may be described as osteolytic or osteoblastic. Osteolytic lesions are characterised by bone destruction due to osteoclast activity while osteoblastic lesions contain new bone produced by osteoblasts. Radionuclide bone scans (Fig. 1) rely on the uptake of technetium in areas of new bone formation to detect metastatic lesions. The purely lytic lesions characteristic of multiple myeloma may not be visualised on bone scan. Prostate cancer is typically associated with osteoblastic lesions.

Bisphosphonates

Bisphosphonates inhibit osteoclast activity. Pamidronate and zoledronic

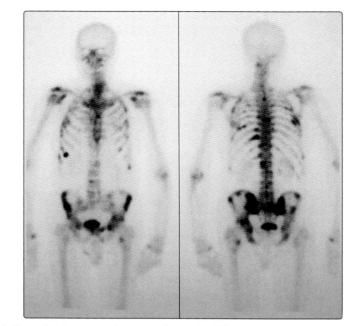

Fig. 1 **Radionuclide bone scan demonstrating multiple bone metastases.** This is a super scan – the kidneys, which are usually seen, are not visualised as all of the radionuclide injected is taken up by the metastatic bone lesions.

acid, which are administered intravenously every 4 weeks, are proven to reduce bone pain, decrease the incidence of fractures and diminish the need for palliative radiotherapy in patients with bone metastases. Renal function should be monitored as nephrotic syndrome is a potential complication. Oral equivalents such as clodronate are also available. Bisphosphonates have not been shown to prevent bone metastases or improve survival.

Radiotherapy

Pain which is localised to the site of a bone lesion can be effectively treated with a single 8 Gy fraction of external beam radiotherapy. This gives pain relief in the majority of cases and can be repeated if pain recurs. Patients with diffuse bone metastases that cannot be encompassed in a standard radiation field may benefit from hemibody irradiation or treatment with a radionuclide. Strontium and samarium emit beta particles which deliver a dose of radiation over a very short distance. Pain which is localised to an area showing uptake on a diagnostic radionuclide scan responds well to a therapeutic radionuclide.

Surgery

Surgical intervention is an effective means of pain control in specific situations such as fracture of the long bones or instability of the spine. Surgery may also be indicated in the management of spinal cord compression.

Brain metastases

Metastatic lesions are the commonest form of intracranial malignancy in adults. Up to one third of adults with cancer will develop brain metastases at some point during the course of their illness. Breast and lung cancer are commonly associated with brain metastases. The majority of lesions occur in the cerebral hemispheres.

Any patient with a known history of cancer presenting with new neurological signs should be investigated for brain metastases. Neurological symptoms and signs associated with intracranial malignancy are discussed in the chapter on primary central nervous system tumours. Most brain metastases can be diagnosed on contrast-enhanced CT. MRI is more sensitive and will help to differentiate metastatic lesions from benign processes when the diagnosis is in doubt. A single brain lesion may require a biopsy to confirm the diagnosis. Multiple lesions characteristic of metastases generally do not require a biopsy.

The prognosis for the majority of patients is very poor once brain metastases have been diagnosed. Palliative treatment with steroids and external beam radiotherapy will relieve symptoms and may extend median survival. Prognosis is frequently determined by the overall burden of disease. A small group of patients suitable for an aggressive treatment approach involving surgical resection and radiotherapy may attain prolonged survival times.

Corticosteroids

Symptom relief within 24 to 48 hours can be achieved with administration of corticosteroids.

Radiotherapy

Palliative radiotherapy to the whole brain is a well-established mode of treatment producing symptomatic improvement in the majority of patients. A wide variety of fractionation schemes are used depending on the performance status of the patient. Patients with a better prognosis may be treated with a smaller dose per fraction to avoid late side effects.

Radiosurgery describes a process which delivers a high dose of radiation to a precisely focused area, which should be less than 3 or 4 cm in size. This can be achieved by modifying a linear accelerator to deliver a thin beam from multiple positions calculated to produce the dose required at the focal point or by using a circular array of radiation sources.

Surgery

A patient with a single brain metastasis against a background of a good performance status and controlled extracranial disease may benefit from surgical resection of the brain metastasis followed by radiotherapy.

Lung metastases

Metastatic disease within the lung may take the form of discrete tumours (Fig. 2) or present as lymphangitis carcinomatosis. The latter is an infiltrative process producing reticular shadows on chest radiograph. Cough, shortness of breath, chest pain and haemoptysis are all common symptoms.

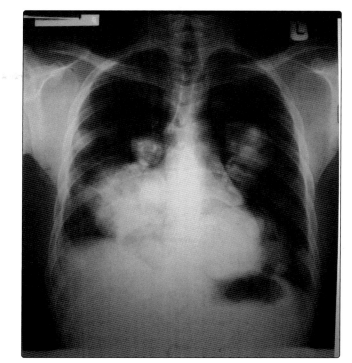

Fig. 2 **Metastatic disease in the lung.**

Supportive therapy includes corticosteroids, antibiotics in the event of intercurrent infection and attention to optimising therapy in patients with pre-existing lung conditions such as chronic obstructive airways disease. Radiotherapy is useful for palliation of pain and haemoptysis. It may also improve shortness of breath caused by a focal obstruction but is unlikely to improve shortness of breath caused by lymphangitis carcinomatosis.

Surgical resection of lung metastases may be indicated in certain conditions, e.g. colorectal carcinoma and sarcoma. In carefully selected patients, resection of metastatic disease in the lung may result in long-term survival.

Liver metastases

Breast, lung and colorectal cancer are common causes of liver metastases. The liver has considerable reserve of function; metastatic disease may not become symptomatic until the disease burden is significant (Fig. 3). Nausea, vomiting, anorexia and right upper quadrant pain due to stretching of the liver capsule may occur. Irritation of the diaphragm with pain referred to the point of the right shoulder is a

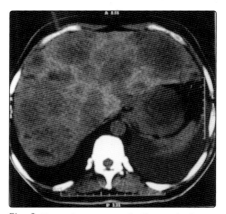

Fig. 3 **Extensive metastatic disease in the liver.**

classic symptom. Jaundice may occur due to widespread disease or localised disease which obstructs the major bile ducts. Symptoms of liver failure herald extensive metastatic disease.

Resection of liver metastases is well established as an effective means of achieving long-term survival in suitable patients with metastatic colorectal cancer. Suitable patients have metastatic disease limited to the liver with controlled or resectable extrahepatic disease. Injection of chemotherapeutic agents directly into the hepatic artery is under investigation.

Specific metastatic conditions

- Appropriate cytotoxic treatment should be considered for metastatic disease.
- Bisphosphonates reduce the incidence of pathological fracture in patients with bone metastases.
- Resection of liver metastases allows long-term survival in suitable patients with colorectal cancer.
- A multidisciplinary approach should be adopted to achieve the best possible quality of life for individual patients.

End of life issues

It should always be possible for terminally ill patients to die without unnecessary pain, anxiety or fear. The task of helping patients transition from active therapy to the palliative phase of care and finally the process of dying can be extremely difficult. It is important that patients' traditions, religion, cultural and spiritual influences are taken into consideration in guiding interactions and end of life care. Communication is an essential tool in the management of patients and their family with regard to end of life issues.

Communication

Research has shown that ideal communication requires careful adjustment of one's approach on an individual by individual basis. An essential prerequisite of efficient communication is to understand that both doctor and patients have their own perspective. As individuals, we are moulded by our experiences, education and available information; these experiences allow us to form our own perspective. Ideal communication accepts that while we do not have direct access to the other's perspective it is essential to develop a feeling of mutual understanding.

It is equally important to comprehend the need to communicate information in a manner that is clear and can be understood from a patient's perspective. As an expert, a doctor has the education and past experiences which allow an understanding of the information and its relevance. The patient on receipt of this information does not have the background, therefore the patient receives the information in a very different frame of reference – it is imperative to know what is the patient's perspective. What do they know? How much do they want to know? Do they understand the importance or relevance of this information?

Although not often possible in the management of a busy oncology service, communication has certain basic requirements:

- Time and attention: it is important to give patients personal time; they must believe there are no other demands on the physician, that they are the focus, and that the physician has time to listen. A physician should turn off all pagers or mobile phones.
- Space: communication can often only be facilitated in a 'safe place', a room where privacy and confidentiality can be assured.

There are certain mechanisms to ideal communication:

- Present the information in clear and understandable language for the patient.
- Bad news is bad news – there is no way to make it better.
- Expand on details only if the patient understands the basic general concept.
- Repeat information.
- Ask the patient what they understand of the given information.

Home care considerations

Caring for a patient at home places increased demands on a family. There are many factors that need to be addressed when determining whether a spouse or family member can handle home care, assuming the primary caregiver role.

- the caregiver's health and motivation, and other demands
- the degree of patient distress
- the technical nature of care
- access to health care.

As an illness progresses, the need for consistent personnel who know the patient's situation becomes the key component of successful delivery of care in the home.

End of life decisions

Ideally, end of life decisions are made early, before there is an urgent need. These issues are difficult to talk to patients about and often entail understanding a patient's philosophical, moral, religious or spiritual background. It is necessary for the health care team and family members to be aware of patients' wishes in order for them to be carried out. Patients don't want to worry families, families don't want to upset patients and unless communication channels remain open, situations may become particularly awkward. A conspiracy of silence can lead to a lonely, isolated death.

A very important decision is whether or not to choose home or hospice care as an alternative to a hospital setting. Whether at home or in hospital, it remains crucial to have access to high-quality palliative care and pain management. Many faith traditions place emphasis on the importance of conscious preparation for death as a way of showing respect for and acceptance of life's final adventure. Getting one's affairs in order also includes working through deep emotions with friends and loved ones, including dealing with grief and bereavement. There are also practical issues around planning funeral or memorial arrangements and settling estates.

Palliative care

The role of palliative care teams are extremely important; it affirms life and regards death as a normal process, but this normal process can be aided by control of physical, psychosocial and spiritual problems.

The NICE clinical guidance on supportive and palliative care advises those who develop and deliver cancer services for adults with cancer. It outlines what is required to ensure that patients, and their families and carers, are well informed, cared for and supported.

The key recommendations are:

- People affected by cancer should be involved in developing cancer services.
- There should be good communication, and people affected by cancer should be involved in decision making.
- Information should be available free of charge.
- People affected by cancer should be offered a range of physical, emotional, spiritual and social support.
- There should be services to help people living with the after-effects of cancer manage these for themselves.
- People with advanced cancer should have access to a range of services to improve their quality of life.

- There should be support for people dying from cancer.
- The needs of family and other carers of people with cancer should be met.
- There should be a trained workforce to provide services.

The Royal College of Physicians (RCP) has issued guidelines, similar to those of the World Health Organization, on the qualities of good palliative care. These appear simpler but are more specific:

- holistic approach to a patient's needs
- relief of symptoms
- extension of care beyond patients to families
- emphasis on quality of life
- good communication
- strong multidisciplinary teamwork.

Symptom control

The qualities outlined by the RCP are all interlinked; a holistic approach to patients' needs implies an emphasis on quality of life and focuses on relief of symptoms. Some of the fears associated with death and dying are uncontrolled pain or other symptoms.

The groundwork for care in the last few days of life should be in the weeks or months preceding. Distressing acute terminal events such as massive haemorrhage or airway obstruction are rare. They can often be anticipated and the patient, the carers and the professional can plan ahead to minimise distress.

The aims of treatment are to:

- reduce pain
- reduce fear
- reduce the level of awareness of the patient.

The event is frightening and distressing for everyone (patients, carers and professionals). Since most such events cause death within minutes, the most important aspect of care is for someone to stay with the patient. The principles of management of most distressing acute terminal events are similar irrespective of the type of event or the cause.

Terminally ill children and palliative care

Age is no barrier to the application of the principles of palliative care; however, it is conceptually more difficult for health care workers, families and children to accept the process of death and dying in a child.

A child with cancer is considered to be moving to palliative care when the child can no longer be treated successfully with available therapies. There may be a long delay between the moment the physician determines the child will not be cured and when everyone agrees that a child has entered the final phase of life.

Important components of the health care team include not only the hospital nurses, physicians, dieticians, therapists but also the family physician. The extended health care team, parents and the family physician should all be involved in the decision-making process from the very beginning of treatment throughout the disease course and at the point of transition to the terminal phase. Depending on the age and level of understanding, the child should also be involved. The child should know as much as possible and appropriate in the situation. In the situation where a child clearly does not wish to be informed of details, their wishes should be respected. Inevitably conflicts may arise with parents' wishes to follow a specific treatment plan which may not be medically or ethically reasonable for a child; however, when the health care team members take time to openly discuss clinical scenarios, conflicts may be resolved. Senseless continuation of aggressive therapy can be detrimental for child, parents and health care team dynamics.

Control of pain, physical and psychological, is of paramount importance at any point in patient management but once a palliative care approach has been embraced it is even more important.

Facilitation of children's wishes to stay at home when possible should be encouraged. Once a child returns home, continued communication with the child, parents and primary health care team should be maintained; follow-up visits and contact with the hospital team should be facilitated to prevent feelings of abandonment developing.

Bereavement counselling should be available after the child's death for the family and siblings. Family members should be encouraged to initiate self-help groups. Parents should be encouraged to discuss with the health care team any issues with the child's care.

Conclusion

Working in health care, with the frequent ravages of cancer and death, results in living with the constant awareness of the impermanence and suffering in life. Knowing the vulnerability of patients with terminal cancer makes them more precious.

As a health care worker dealing with cancer patients and their families it is vital that we adopt measures to cope with the constant stresses of work and life.

End of life issues

- Good communication is essential in the management of patients and their family with regard to end of life issues.
- Communication is facilitated by adequate time and privacy.
- Formation of a multidisciplinary team approach to manage end of life issues is helpful.
- It is imperative to involve the palliative care team at an early stage

Cancer genetics

The vast majority of cancers arise as a result of sporadic genetic mutations in specific cells. Hereditary cancers account for approximately 5–10% of all cancers and are due to germline mutations in genes which predispose to cancer. A germline mutation is present in every cell of the body and may be passed on to the next generation.

Hereditary cancer

A germline mutation in an oncogene, tumour suppressor gene or mismatch repair gene may produce hereditary cancer. The genetic abnormality is referred to as a genotype, while the clinical manifestation is the phenotype. Some examples of known hereditary cancer syndromes are given in Table 1.

- *Oncogenes.* Proto-oncogenes are a normal part of the genome. Mutation produces an oncogene which usually demonstrates a 'gain in function' producing uncontrolled cell growth and proliferation. Inheritance of this type of mutation is usually autosomal dominant. This means that 50% of offspring will inherit the defect.
- *Tumour suppressor genes.* These genes prevent carcinogenesis as the name suggests. Most cancer predisposition genes are tumour suppressor genes. Mutation in these genes results in 'loss of function'

with consequent development of cancer. These genes are usually inherited in a recessive pattern; a mutation must also occur in the normal copy of the gene for cancer to develop.
- *Mismatch repair genes.* This group of genes control elaborate DNA repair mechanisms. This intricate mechanism is required because the complex structure of the DNA is constantly exposed to damage within the nucleus. In addition, the process of DNA duplication produces errors which must be corrected. Mutation of these genes results in an accumulation of DNA damage which may ultimately cause cancer. Inheritance is usually autosomal recessive.

Family history

An accurate family history covering at least three generations will identify a hereditary cancer risk in most cases. The family pedigree should be annotated in standard format (see Fig. 1). The type of cancer and the age at diagnosis should be recorded for all affected individuals. Medical notes or death certificates may be required to confirm the diagnosis, particularly if cancer is reported as 'stomach' or 'abdominal'. Characteristics associated with a potential genetic predisposition are described in Box 1. Knowledge of

Box 1 Indicators of potential genetic predisposition

- Young age at diagnosis
- Multiple primary cancers in one individual
- Cancers in multiple family members
- Clustering of specific cancer types, e.g. breast and ovarian cancer suggest *BRCA1* or *BRCA2* mutations
- Bilateral cancer in paired organs, e.g. bilateral breast cancer
- Association with features of known cancer syndromes, e.g. MEN 1 and 2
- High-risk ethnic group, e.g. Ashkenazi Jewish origin

inherited cancer syndromes and an accurate family tree often allow a specialist to estimate the risk of cancer in a particular individual in the family.

Genetic counselling and testing

Genetic counselling is a well-defined process designed to anticipate the significant psychological and scientific issues which will be encountered by individuals and their families prior to and after a genetic test is performed. Several visits to a specialised counselling service over a period of at least one month are usually required prior to a genetic test actually being done. A typical process is described here.

Table 1 **Examples of hereditary cancer syndromes**				
Syndrome	**Gene**	**Cancer**	**Lifetime risk of cancer**	**Risk reduction strategies**
Breast and ovarian cancer	*BRCA1*	Breast	50–80%	Offer genetic testing
		Ovary	20–40%	*For affected family members:*
		Colon	6%	Screen from 30 years of age or start 5 years before the age at which the
		Prostate	5%	youngest case was diagnosed
				Screening tests:
	BRCA2	Breast	50–80%	■ Breast examination, mammography and breast MRI
		Ovary	30%	■ Annual transvaginal ultrasound
		Prostate	15%	■ Annual CA125
		Male breast cancer	5%	*Consider:*
		Pancreas		Prophylactic bilateral mastectomy
		Melanoma		Prophylactic oophorectomy
		Others		
Familial adenomatous polyposis (FAP)	*APC*	Colon	100%	Offer genetic testing
		Stomach		*For affected family members:*
		Duodenal ampulla		Prophylactic total colectomy
		Thyroid		
Hereditary non-polyposis colorectal cancer (HNPCC)				
Lynch type 1	*hMSH2*	Colon	70%	Offer genetic testing
Lynch type 2	*hMLH1*	Colon	70%	*For affected family members:*
	hMLH6	Endometrium	Up to 40%	Screen from age 25 upwards, or 5 younger than youngest case in family
	hPMS1	Ovary	Up to 20%	■ Annual colonoscopy
	hPMS2	Others		■ Annual pelvic/transvaginal ultrasound
	hMLH3			■ Annual CA125

At the time of referral, an individual is given information on hereditary predisposition to cancer. The family history is documented in as much detail as possible and the individual's risk of carrying a genetic mutation is discussed. The second visit is initiated by the individual. The benefits and limitations of genetic testing as well as the potential impact of both positive and negative test results are discussed. The issue of disclosure of results to family members is considered at this stage. A positive genetic test may cause severe personal and familial psychological morbidity and have far-reaching financial implications. Genetic testing is performed at a third visit if desired. Support, advice and recommendations regarding risk reduction strategies are provided as necessary.

The available data on genetic predisposition to cancer are complex and constantly changing as progress is made. However, the investigative process is based on a few key questions listed here and discussed with reference to Fig. 1.

1. Does the family carry a gene predisposing to cancer?

The family history may indicate that a particular cancer syndrome is highly likely. Fig. 1 illustrates a pedigree which suggests the presence of a mutation in *BRCA1* or *BRCA2*, details of which are given in Table 1.

2. Does this individual carry the gene?

The risk that an individual carries a familial cancer gene is approximately 50% in the case of autosomal dominant inheritance. Ideally, diagnostic and predictive DNA analysis will give a definitive answer. However, there are many cancer syndromes for which there is no clinical test available or which may be caused by multiple gene mutations. In the absence of an available test, an estimation of risk is made by a specialist based on the available clinical information. In this case, there is a test available for *BRCA1* and *BRCA2* mutations.

Diagnostic testing

An *affected* family member is tested for known cancer-causing mutations in a specific gene, e.g. *BRCA1* and *BRCA2*. A negative test does not rule out the possibility of a genetic predisposition. It may occur in the following cases:

- The causative gene may not yet be known. *BRCA1* and *BRCA2* account for approximately 60% of familial breast cancer.
- No test is available for the causative gene.
- Inaccurate family history may lead to testing for the wrong gene.
- Technical reasons, e.g. the test is not 100% sensitive.

Predictive testing

An *unaffected* family member is tested for a known mutation to ascertain whether he or she is a carrier. Predictive testing can only be performed if a cancer-causing gene has been identified in an affected family member. If the unaffected family member tests negative for the identified mutation, the risk of cancer for that individual becomes the same as for the general population.

3. What is the risk of this individual developing cancer?

The risk of cancer in someone carrying a *BRCA1* or *BRCA2* mutation is reasonably well documented (Table 1). Databases of families with high-risk histories or known cancer-causing mutations provide information which allows calculation of the risk of cancer for people with similar histories or mutations. The risk of cancer is often quoted as a lifetime risk or the risk of developing cancer by a certain age. Various mathematical models have been devised to assist in individual risk estimation. For less common familial cancer syndromes, reliable risk estimation is very difficult due to the paucity of clinical information.

Case study

Mary is 45 years of age and has just completed adjuvant treatment for right-sided breast cancer. Her family history is illustrated in Fig. 1. Mary has two daughters aged 12 and 13 and is concerned about their risk of cancer. Mary undergoes genetic counselling and is tested for *BRCA1* and *BRCA2* mutations.

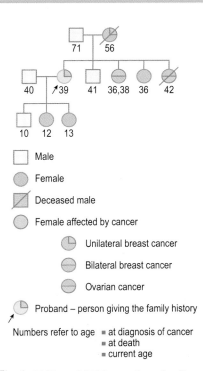

Fig. 1 **BRCA1 or BRCA2 mutation – family pedigree.**

Outcome 1

Mary's test is positive for a *BRCA1* mutation known to cause cancer. This gene is inherited in an autosomal dominant manner, which means that each of her daughters has a 50% chance of having the gene. Being a carrier confers a substantial risk of developing cancer in adulthood. Ideally, the children should be allowed to make their own decision regarding genetic testing when they reach adulthood.

Outcome 2

Mary's test is negative for *BRCA1* and *BRCA2* mutations. Given the family history, it is highly likely that a genetic predisposition is present but has not been identified. Mary's daughters would have to be considered at high risk until further information becomes available. Breast cancer is a common disease; therefore it is also possible that Mary's breast cancer represents a phenocopy – a sporadic case occurring in a family with a genetic predisposition. In this case, testing Mary's sister may reveal the genetic predisposition.

Cancer genetics

- 5–10% of cancers are hereditary.
- Hereditary cancer may be caused by a germline mutation in oncogenes, tumour suppressor genes or mismatch repair genes.
- Genetic counselling and testing is an intricate process carried out in a specialised clinic.
- Many familial cancer syndromes confer a high lifetime risk of cancer.

- Various risk reduction strategies may be employed in specific situations.
- *Key questions:*
  - □ Does the family carry a gene predisposing to cancer?
  - □ Does this individual carry the gene?
  - □ What is this individual's risk of cancer?

Late effects of treatment

Both chemotherapy and radiotherapy are associated with significant long-term side effects. As cancer treatment outcomes have improved, particularly in the paediatric field, the number of long-term cancer survivors is increasing. Late side effects must be taken into account when deciding optimal treatment for patients who are likely to be long-term survivors. For example, radiotherapy is to be delivered with caution in the treatment of young women with early stage Hodgkin's disease as it is associated with a significant increase in breast cancer and other solid tumours. Fifteen years after treatment for Hodgkin's disease, the mortality from treatment-related side effects such as second malignancy and pulmonary and cardiac damage exceeds the mortality from Hodgkin's disease.

The late effects of cancer treatment may not become apparent for some time. Leukaemia and lymphomas may occur after 5 to 10 years. Secondary solid tumours tend to manifest after 10 to 20 years. Damage to specific organs may manifest over a variable period of time depending on the treatment given and the function of the organ prior to treatment. Accurate data collection requires follow-up over extended periods of time.

Chemotherapy and radiotherapy may have synergistic adverse effects if toxicity profiles overlap. For example, pneumonitis due to irradiation of lung tissue will compound lung damage due to the administration of bleomycin.

Radiotherapy

Ionising radiation is indiscriminate and will affect all tissues in the path of the beam. The converse is also true – the radiation beam does not affect organs outside the radiation field. Late side effects are defined as those occurring ≥90 days after treatment, although effects may not become apparent for many years. The clinical manifestations vary according to the organ involved (Table 1).

Historically, late side effects were thought to be progressive and irreversible due to loss of specific cell populations or damage to the microvasculature. It is now understood that cytokine-mediated cascades inducing inflammatory and fibrotic responses play an important part in the development of late reactions.

Variables affecting the occurrence of late side effects of radiotherapy

Patient variables
- Age at the time of treatment.
- Pre-treatment organ function.
- Tumour-related organ damage.
- Radiosensitivity of the individual – sensitivity to radiation varies among patients receiving the same treatment. Certain conditions are known to increase the risk of side effects, e.g. active collagen vascular disease, inflammatory bowel disease and smoking.
- Rare genetic disorders associated with increased radiation sensitivity, e.g. ataxia telangiectasia.

Treatment variables
- Total dose – increasing the total dose increases the likelihood of late side effects. Current and previous radiotherapy treatments must be taken into account when assessing the total dose.
- Dose per fraction – exceeding the conventional 2 Gy per fraction increases the risk of late side effects.

For this reason, large fractions are usually reserved for palliative treatments, when the risk of late side effects is of reduced clinical importance.
- Overall treatment time – shortening the overall treatment time may be associated with increased late side effects.
- The volume of the organ treated – an organ such as the lung may tolerate a high dose to a small volume without compromising organ function, while a low dose to the entire organ will cause significant clinical symptoms.
- Radiosensitivity of the organ treated – innate sensitivity to radiotherapy varies among tissues. For example, the lens of the eye will develop a cataract after 6 Gy while the retina may withstand 50 Gy without impairment of function.
- Chemotherapy:
  - administration of concomitant chemotherapy
  - previous treatment with chemotherapeutic agents causing specific organ toxicities.

Dose–volume histograms
Three-dimensional conformal radiotherapy planning uses CT images to outline the normal organs at risk. The normal organs at risk are those which may receive a portion of the prescribed radiation dose. For instance, the normal organs at risk in the treatment of lung cancer would include the normal lung tissue, heart, spinal cord and oesophagus.

A dose–volume histogram is a graph of dose versus volume of the organ, used by the radiation oncologist to help choose the optimal treatment plan. Dose constraints can be applied to reduce the potential for side effects to acceptable levels, e.g. the maximum dose to the spinal cord should not exceed 50 Gy delivered at 2 Gy per fraction. A dose–volume histogram is illustrated in Fig. 1.

Chemotherapy

Chemotherapeutic agents may produce a wide spectrum of side effects. Individual drugs are associated with specific toxicity profiles, e.g. high-dose cyclophosphamide may cause

Table 1 **Late side effects of radiotherapy**	
Organ	**Late effects**
Spinal cord	Transverse myelitis
Brain	Impairment of memory and concentration, somnolence syndrome, necrosis, diffuse white matter injury (Fig. 2)
Lung	Pneumonitis, fibrosis
Heart	Cardiomyopathy, constrictive pericarditis, coronary artery disease, conduction defects
Bowel	Stenosis, obstruction, fistula formation, perforation, haemorrhage
Reproductive system	Women – menopause, infertility, impaired sexual function
	Men – infertility, impaired sexual function
Skin	Telangiectasia (Fig. 3), fibrosis, atrophy

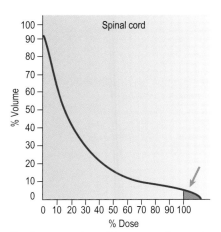

Fig. 1 **Dose–volume histogram.** The spinal cord will tolerate a radiation dose of 50 Gy with acceptably low risk of late side effects. This dose–volume histogram shows that a small proportion of the cord will receive more than 100% of the dose (arrow); 50 Gy cannot be administered safely based on this treatment plan – the dose must be reduced or the treatment plan revised.

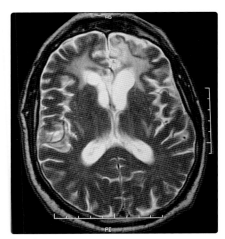

Fig. 2 **Appearance of the brain on MRI** 3 years after radiotherapy to the frontal lobes.

haemorrhagic cystitis due to an active metabolite called acrolein accumulating in the bladder.

Variables affecting the occurrence of side effects after chemotherapy

Patient variables
- The age of the patient at the time of treatment; for example, combination chemotherapy is more likely to induce menopause in perimenopausal women.
- Pre-treatment organ function.
- Tumour-related organ damage.
- Specific conditions; for example, a rare disorder resulting in

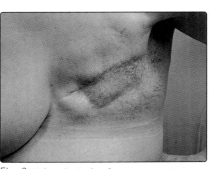

Fig. 3 **Telangiectasia after post-mastectomy radiotherapy.**

reduced levels of the enzyme dihydropyrimidine dehydrogenase is associated with markedly increased toxicity with 5-fluorouracil.

Treatment variables
- The cumulative lifetime dose administered is a risk factor for the clinical appearance of side effects. This has led to lifetime threshold dose recommendations. An alternative approach is to establish baseline organ function and monitor subsequent function at frequent intervals during treatment. This approach requires a good knowledge of the natural history of organ damage caused by the drug, which should include an early, treatable stage amenable to diagnosis by the screening test.
- Administration of agents with overlapping toxicity profiles; for example, doxorubicin and trastuzumab, which are both potentially cardiotoxic, may be given in the treatment of breast cancer.
- Concomitant administration of radiotherapy.

Adult survivors of childhood cancer

As the outlook for children with cancer improves, the number of adult survivors of childhood cancer is growing. The administration of chemotherapeutic agents or radiation therapy during childhood may have detrimental effects on immature tissues. This group of patients is prone to specific medical, psychological and social long-term problems, some of which are mentioned below. Follow-up is hugely important and should ideally be lifelong to facilitate collection of

accurate data and timely treatment of emerging late side effects.

Long-term side effects
- Growth failure may occur as a consequence of radiotherapy to the brain, spine or growth centres. Hormone deficiency (i.e. growth hormone/thyroid hormone), chronic illness and complex psychological issues also contribute. It may not be possible to pinpoint a specific cause.
- Infertility – radiotherapy and many chemotherapeutic drugs may result in sterility in both males and females. Age-appropriate advice regarding the use of facilities such as sperm banking should be given. Infertility due to radiotherapy should be avoided by moving the ovaries or testes out of the radiation field prior to treatment.
- Education and employment – prolonged illness impacts directly on school attendance. In addition, treatments such as cranial irradiation in young children are associated with reduced IQ and inability to take on full-time independent employment in adulthood.
- Risk of second malignancy – studies of patients treated for Hodgkin's disease have found an increased risk of leukaemias and non-Hodgkin's lymphoma 5 to 10 years after chemotherapy and radiotherapy. Solid tumours such as lung and breast cancer are related to radiotherapy treatment fields. Survival after occurrence of second malignancy is poor.

Late effects of treatment
- As cancer treatments improve, the number of long-term cancer survivors is increasing.
- Surgery, radiotherapy and chemotherapy may all produce significant long-term side effects.
- Patients treated for Hodgkin's disease demonstrate an increased increased risk of leukaemia, lymphoma and solid tumours after treatment with chemotherapy and radiotherapy.
- Mortality due to long-term side effects exceeds mortality due to Hodgkin's disease 15 years after treatment.

Pregnancy and cancer

Cancer associated with pregnancy is unusual; the estimated incidence is 1 in 1000 pregnancies. It has become more common in the last 30 years because of the increasing number of women pregnant at older age. However, because of the relative rareness of this association, there is a paucity of information on the effects of the disease and its therapy on pregnancy outcome.

When cancer occurs in pregnancy, there is frequently a conflict between optimal maternal therapy and fetal well-being. Cancer is the second leading cause of death in women during their reproductive years. It constitutes a difficult clinical situation, dealing with issues of both maternal well-being and fetal prognosis.

Chemotherapy in pregnancy

Cytotoxic chemotherapy causes genetic damage in exposed somatic cells, including chromosomal breaks, translocations, deletions, gene mutations, aneuploidy and cell cycle disruption. Most cytotoxic drugs have a molecular weight less than 600 kDa, and can cross the placenta and reach the embryonal circulation, unless they are extensively bound to plasma proteins.

During the first 2–4 weeks from conception, cell differentiation and organogenesis are minimal. Later in the first trimester of pregnancy, chemotherapy may interfere with organogenesis, with the risk of teratogenesis being maximal. During the second and third trimesters organogenesis is complete with the exception of the CNS and gonads. Fetal ultrasound can accurately assess age and thus can be used to assess risk of therapy at a defined time (Fig. 1).

Radiation in pregnancy

The developing embryo and fetus are extremely sensitive to ionising radiation, which might cause pregnancy loss, malformations, growth retardation and neurobehavioural defects. The effects of exposure are dose and time dependent. There is a paucity of research on the long-term neurological and behavioural development of children exposed to radiation in utero.

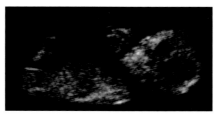

Fig. 1 **A week 10 fetus in a patient presenting with a breast lump.**

Analysis of the data of survivors from Hiroshima and Nagasaki demonstrated that the highest risk of brain damage occurred between 8 and 15 weeks of gestational age. The apparent absence of an effect prior to the eighth week suggests that neuronal cell migration during weeks 8–15 post conception may be the crucial component of cerebral damage caused by radiation.

Specific cancers in pregnancy

Cervical cancer

This is one the commonest cancers of pregnancy, affecting 1 in 2000 pregnancies. Around 1–5% of patients with cervical cancer are diagnosed while pregnant. The majority of patients are asymptomatic and diagnosed by abnormal cytology perhaps due to the frequent gynaecological examination. All suspicious lesions should be biopsied. Risks are outlined in Table 1. When indicated, conisation should be performed between 14 and 20 weeks.

Staging consists of physical examination, chest X-ray and MRI of abdomen/pelvis. Pathological findings do not differ in the pregnant patient; the majority of cases are squamous cell carcinomas.

Stage Ia

- First trimester <3 mm depth of invasion: delay therapy until after delivery vaginally.
- 3–5 mm depth of invasion and/or lymphatic/vascular invasion: deliver by caesarean section as soon as fetal maturity is reached.
- Second or third trimester defer therapy. Radical treatment may follow postpartum.

Stage Ib–IV

- First or second trimester: pregnancy termination and immediate

institution of therapy is traditionally advised. Studies to date have not shown adverse maternal outcomes after treatment delays of 5–40 weeks.
- Third trimester: deferral of therapy until after delivery by caesarean section, weeks 32–36, is possible.

Little data exist examining the safety of caesarean section versus vaginal delivery. But the risks of obstructed labour, haemorrhage and episiotomy site recurrence with vaginal delivery have led to the recommendation of caesarean delivery. Cervical cancer does not appear to affect the outcome of pregnancy. Laser vaporisation of the uterine cervix does not influence the outcome of subsequent pregnancy.

Breast cancer

This occurs in 1 in 3000 pregnancies, the average patient being 32–38 years. It is defined as a cancer diagnosed during or up to 12 months postpartum. The most common presentation is a painless palpable lump. Breast cancer pathology is similar in age-matched women.

To detect breast cancer, pregnant and lactating women should practise self-examination and undergo a breast examination as part of the routine prenatal examination by a doctor. If an abnormality is found, ultrasound or shielded mammography may be used. Since at least 25% of mammograms in pregnancy may be negative in the presence of cancer, a biopsy is essential with any palpable mass.

- *Stage I/II*. Modified radical mastectomy and axillary node dissection or conservative surgery with postpartum radiation therapy has been used. Adjuvant chemotherapy should be avoided in the first trimester; certain agents may be considered in the second or third trimester such as

Table 1 **Risks of cervical biopsy in pregnant patient**	
Colposcopy directed biopsy	
Haemorrhage	1–3%
Conisation or loop excision biopsy	
Vaginal bleeding	5–15%
Abortion	25%
Infection	15%
Premature delivery	15%
Residual disease	30–50%

CMF (cyclophosphamide, methotrexate, 5-fluorouracil), AC (Adriamycin, cyclophosphamide), CAF (cyclophosphamide, Adriamycin, 5-fluorouracil) with only a 1.3% risk of malformation. Data on taxanes are limited.

■ *Stage III/IV*. Surgery can proceed as clinically indicated. Radiation should be deferred until postpartum while chemotherapy options are similar to above – avoid chemotherapy in the first trimester unless termination of pregnancy is planned; one could consider certain chemotherapies in the second and third trimester, although data are still limited.

Melanoma

Melanoma constitutes 8% of malignancies diagnosed during pregnancy, 1 in 1000–10 000 pregnancies. Most arise from pre-existing naevi; changes in size, colour and configuration of any pigmented lesions should raise suspicion. Normal pregnancy-related hyperpigmentation may lead to diagnosis delay. Excisional biopsy is the recommended procedure.

Staging investigations chosen depend on the clinical suspicion and stage of pregnancy. Sentinel node dissection for those with worrisome clinical features should use the 'blue-dye' rather than radiolabelled technique.

■ Surgical removal of the melanoma with adequate margins remains the standard primary therapy for early melanoma.
■ Adjuvant interferon therapy should be deferred until postpartum.
■ Management of metastatic melanoma is palliative.

Malignant melanoma is the tumour that most frequently metastasises to the placenta or fetus. Therefore, the placenta should be thoroughly examined for metastasis. If present, the infant should be monitored for development of malignant disease.

Lymphoma

Since Hodgkin's lymphoma affects primarily young adults, most oncologists will eventually face the dilemma of how to provide therapy to a pregnant woman while minimising the risk to the fetus. However, non-Hodgkin's lymphoma (NHL) may also present in the pregnant patient. Most patients present with painless lymphadenopathy (70–80%) while only

one fifth have 'B' symptoms. The presenting stage, clinical behaviour, prognosis, and histological subtypes of Hodgkin's lymphoma during pregnancy do not differ from those of non-pregnant women during their childbearing years.

Staging should include bone marrow aspiration/biopsy, chest X-ray, abdominopelvic ultrasound or MRI and laboratory work-up. Nodular sclerosis is the most common Hodgkin's lymphoma histology, while gestational NHL is usually high grade such as B-diffuse large cell lymphoma, Burkitt-like or B-lymphoblastic.

■ Early stage – patients can be followed carefully with plans to induce delivery early and proceed with definitive therapy. Alternatively, these patients can receive radiation therapy with proper shielding.
■ In the event of a first trimester diagnosis in a patient with B symptoms, advanced stage, bulky stage or evidence of aggressive disease, termination of pregnancy and initiation of therapy must be considered.
■ In the second and third trimesters, the relative safety of therapy has been demonstrated with a stillbirth risk of 4% and miscarriage 10%.
■ Third trimester births may be managed expectantly with induction of delivery at 32 to 36 weeks and then postpartum chemotherapy.

Other cancers

Ovarian cancer, leukaemias, colorectal cancer, gastric cancer, thyroid cancer and non-small cell lung cancer have all been described in the literature. These cancers occur with increasing rarity.

Placental and fetal metastases

Vertical transmission of malignant cells to the placenta or fetus is

uncommon. Seeding may occur as a result of haematogenous spread, lymphatic spread or contiguous invasion (pelvic tumours).

The most common cancers involved are:

■ melanoma (32%)
■ leukaemia/lymphoma (15%)
■ breast (13%)
■ gastric (3%)
■ lung/gynaecological (3%).

Macroscopic and histopathological examination of the placenta with meticulous study of the intravillous spaces and villi should be routinely done in every case of malignancy coexisting with pregnancy.

Breastfeeding

Breastfeeding is usually not recommended during maternal therapy with anticancer chemotherapy. This is because the dose-dependent and dose-independent effects of these drugs are not completely understood.

Clinical studies in this area are particularly scarce; Table 2 documents the available information.

Table 2 **Drugs and breastfeeding**	
Drug	**Data**
Cisplatin	Conflicting data
Cyclophosphamide	Distributed in breast milk as documented neutropenia in breastfed children
Doxorubicin	Preclinical studies show metabolite present in low quantities, but no clinical data
Methotrexate	No data
Antiemetics	Domperidone and metoclopramide are excreted into milk in a small amount. No adverse effect on the infant has been reported
Allopurinol	Although a metabolite may be detected in the infant's plasma after breastfeeding, no adverse effect has been reported
Azathioprine	Small quantities are found in breast milk, but in two reports breastfed infants showed no sign of toxicity. Some experts recommend formula feeding because of inherent toxicity of the drug

Pregnancy and cancer

■ Cancer diagnosed during pregnancy is a dramatic event with profound impact on the lives of the patient, family and offspring.
■ It is rare, with an estimated incidence of 1 in 1000 pregnancies.
■ Cervical, breast and melanoma are the most common.
■ Placental and fetal metastases have been documented rarely.

Paraneoplastic syndromes

Paraneoplastic syndromes occur in 10–20% of patients. They represent a wide range of disease entities as a result of non-metastatic effects of cancer. They may either pre- or post-date the diagnosis of cancer, and result in significant morbidity. In general, they may respond to therapy directed at the underlying malignancy.

Many paraneoplastic conditions have been described (Table 1); however, we shall concentrate on the more common syndromes.

Mechanism of action

The relationship between the syndrome and underlying malignancy is very complex. The syndromes are believed to be caused by the production of a variety of substances by the tumour:

- antibodies
- hormones
- protein hormone precursors
- enzymes
- fetal proteins
- cytokines.

General paraneoplastic symptoms

Fever, night sweats anorexia, cachexia arise from the release of lymphokines involved in the immune response or mediators of tumour cell death such as tumour necrosis factor alpha (TNFα), IL-1, IL-6 and interferon.

Paraneoplastic neurological disorders

Paraneoplastic neurological disorders (PNDs) are rare syndromes caused by an immune response against onconeural antigens. These antigens are common to both normal neural tissue and tumour. The presence of autoantibodies (Table 2) establishes the diagnosis of PND.

The most common PND is a peripheral neuropathy producing mild motor weakness, sensory loss and absent distal reflexes. It may be due to nutritional deprivation but responds poorly to nutritional therapy. A rare variant subacute sensory neuropathy consists of dorsal root ganglia degeneration and progressive sensory loss with ataxia. Diagnosis is made with the clinical features and presence of anti-Hu in the serum of some patients with lung cancer.

The Eaton–Lambert syndrome is an immune-mediated, myasthenia-like syndrome with weakness usually affecting the limbs and sparing ocular and bulbar muscles. It is caused by an IgG antibody (anti-VGCC) causing impaired nerve terminal release of acetylcholine. It occurs most commonly with SCLC (70%). Diagnosis is confirmed with electromyography (EMG) studies and anti-VGCC present. Treatment is first directed at the underlying malignancy. Guanidine, corticosteroids or plasmapheresis may be beneficial.

Subacute cerebellar degeneration causes progressive bilateral leg and arm ataxia, dysarthria, and sometimes vertigo and diplopia with rapid progression. This disease is most commonly found in SCLC, ovary, breast and lymphoma. Cerebellar atrophy will be seen on MRI or CT. Anti-Yo, anti-Ri and anti-Hu are all found in this disorder. Treatment is non-specific, but some improvement may follow successful cancer therapy.

Endocrine paraneoplastic syndromes

Syndrome of inappropriate antidiuretic hormone (SIADH) secretion is only found in 3–15% of patients with SCLC, but 75% of cases seen are secondary to SCLC. It is important to note that some chemotherapy agents can cause a transient SIADH – the vinca alkaloids, cyclophosphamide, ifosfamide and cisplatin. The cardinal features are water intoxication and hyponatraemia – decreased serum osmolarity, inappropriately high urine osmolarity with urine sodium >20 meq/L in the setting of normal renal, adrenal and thyroid function. Treatment of the underlying cancer often results in control of the syndrome; supportive measures may be needed while awaiting response. Demeclocycline can effectively normalise sodium levels.

Cushing's syndrome (cortisol excess, leading to hyperglycaemia, hypokalaemia, hypertension, central

Table 1 Paraneoplastic syndromes

Condition	Association
Neurological	
Dermatomyositis/polymyositis	Proximal myopathy, rash, elevated creatine kinase with diagnostic EMG and biopsy, seen with adenocarcinomas
Eaton–Lambert syndrome	Autoimmune progressive weakness and cholinergic symptoms with SCLC
Myasthenia gravis	Autoimmune muscle fatigability usually seen with thymoma
Cerebellar degeneration	Cerebellar signs in SCLC, ovarian and breast cancer patients
Neuropathies	More commonly sensory mononeuritis/polyneuritis associated with SCLC
Encephalitis	Autoimmune condition causing confusion, amnesia in lung cancer patients
Endocrine	
SIADH	Commonly seen with NSCLC
Hypercalcaemia	Multifactorial, common in squamous carcinomas, parathyroid hormone-related peptide
Cushing's syndrome	Ectopic ACTH production
Zollinger–Ellison syndrome	Ectopic gastrin secretion with gastrinomas, MEN type 1
Cutaneous	
Sweet's syndrome	Erythematous plaques of face and neck associated with leucocytosis, such as leukaemias
Tylosis	Thickening of palms and soles associated with oesophageal cancer
Acanthosis nigricans	Velvet appearing skin thickening of axilla, palms, soles, perineum associated with adenocarcinomas
Leser–Trélat syndrome	Multiple seborrhoeic warts seen with GI cancers
Hypertrichosis lanuginosa acquisita	Lanugo hair associated with colon, uterus, lung cancer and lymphoma
Ichthyosis	Dry scaly skin seen with lymphoma, lung, testes and ovarian cancer
Rheumatological	
Hypertrophic pulmonary osteoarthropathy (HPOA)	Clubbing and painful swelling of distal long bones due to new bone formation associated with lung cancer
Vasculitis	May occur with a wide variety of cancers
Gastrointestinal	
Protein losing enteropathy	GI cancers and lymphomas cause oedema, weight loss and hypogammaglobulinaemia

Table 2 **Autoantibodies causing PNDs**

Antibody	Site of action	Clinical syndrome	Cancer
Anti-Hu	Pan-neuronal	Encephalomyelitis, sensory neuropathy, autonomic neuropathy	SCLC, sarcoma, neuroblastoma
Anti-Ri	CNS neurons	Opsiclonus–myoclonus, cerebellar ataxia	Breast, gynaecological, SCLC, bladder
Anti-Yo	Purkinje cell	Cerebellar degeneration	Ovary, uterus, breast, SCLC
Anti-VGCC	Presynaptic neuromuscular junction	Eaton–Lambert syndrome	SCLC, Hodgkin's disease
Anti-CAR	Photoreceptors	Cancer-associated retinopathy	SCLC, melanoma
Anti-Ta	Nucleus	Limbic encephalitis	Testis

obesity, and 'moon facies') may result from ectopic production of ACTH or ACTH-like molecules, most often with SCLC. Medical therapy for ectopic ACTH production involves inhibiting cortisol production. The drug with the most favourable toxicity profile is ketoconazole but other potential agents are mitotane, metyrapone or aminoglutethamide.

Cutaneous paraneoplastic syndromes

A wide variety of cutaneous syndromes are associated with malignancies.

Acanthosis nigricans is characterised by a pruritic symmetrical brown-grey velvety hyperpigmentation found in the neck, axilla, flexor areas and anogenital area. It affects men and women equally and is most often associated with adenocarcinomas of the GI tract, particularly gastric.

Leser–Trélat syndrome is recognised by the presence of multiple seborrhoeic keratoses which are found in elderly patients with gastric adenocarcinoma, lymphoma or breast cancer (Fig. 1).

Sweet's syndrome is associated with fever, neutrophilia and the appearances of erythematous raised cutaneous plaques distributed in the face, neck and upper body. It may be related to cancer in 20% of patients or drug induced (Fig. 2).

Flushing or episodic facial reddening typically lasting minutes is associated with carcinoid syndrome but also seen with leukaemia, medullary carcinoma of thyroid and renal cell carcinoma. This is related to the secretion of vasoactive peptides such as serotonin. Ichthyosis is characterised by generalised cracking skin, hyperkeratotic palms and soles and rhomboidal scales. It is associated with haematological malignancies. Other skin disorders have also been documented such as lichenoid type reactions (Fig. 3).

Fig. 1 **Leser–Trélat syndrome in an elderly man with lymphoma.**

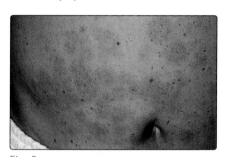
Fig. 2 **Sweet's syndrome in a leukaemic patient receiving G-CSF.**

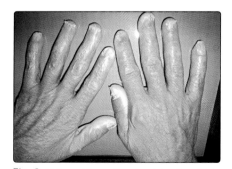
Fig. 3 **Lichenoid reaction** involving the distal digits and nail beds secondary to lymphoproliferative disorder.

Rheumatological paraneoplastic syndromes

Hypertrophic pulmonary osteoarthropathy is a rare disorder that is associated with severe clubbing. It is associated with certain lung cancers.

This disorder is characterised by:

- subperiosteal new bone formation at the distal ends of long bones
- symmetrical arthropathy of adjacent joints

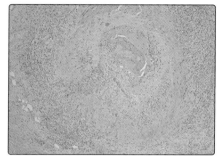
A

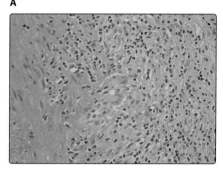
B
Fig. 4 **A patient with multiple myeloma** developed polymyalgia rheumatica with visual symptoms; temporal artery biopsy demonstrated a giant cell arteritis.

- clubbing of the fingers
- gynaecomastia.

Polymyositis/dermatomyositis are more common in patients with cancer, especially in those >50 years. Patients describe progressive proximal muscle weakness. A dusky, erythematous butterfly rash with a heliotrope hue may develop on the cheeks, with periorbital oedema. Vasculitis may occur as part of the spectrum of rheumatological disorders or as a paraneoplastic disorder (Fig. 4).

Paraneoplastic syndromes

- Paraneoplastic disorders occur in 10–20% of patients with cancer, which may pre- or post-date the diagnosis.
- Any body system may be involved.
- It is caused by the production of tumour-related antibodies, hormones, enzymes and cytokines
- Treatment of the underlying cancer is the appropriate management of the disorder.

Immunosuppression and malignancy

HIV/AIDS

The case definition for AIDS was first defined by the Centers for Disease Control in North America in the early 1980s. The inclusion of certain conditions has been the subject of some controversy over the years and the case definition has been revised on several occasions, most recently in 1993 at which time cervical cancer was added. Kaposi's sarcoma, lymphoma and invasive cervical cancer are all considered AIDS-defining illnesses according to this case definition. Other cancers which occur in increased incidence in the HIV-infected population are described as being associated with HIV and are listed in Box 1.

With the advent of highly active anti-retroviral treatment (HAART), people with HIV/AIDS in the developed world are now living longer. HAART reduces the viral load and increases the CD4 count, thus reducing vulnerability to opportunistic infections. As a result, HIV-associated cancers are responsible for an increasing proportion of morbidity and mortality in people with HIV/AIDS.

Kaposi's sarcoma and non-Hodgkin's lymphoma account for most malignancy in HIV-positive patients, their incidence rising sharply when the CD4 count is $<200/\mu L$. It is therefore expected that the widespread use of HAART will reduce the incidence of these conditions. For cervical cancer and HIV-associated cancers there may be no clear-cut association between cancer incidence and the level of immunosuppression as measured by CD4 counts. In the case of cervical cancer, additional factors such as human papilloma virus, smoking and lifestyle also play a role in causation.

Cancer treatment in HIV-positive patients

HIV-positive patients with good performance status can be treated with standard chemotherapeutic drugs and radiotherapy. The toxicity of cancer treatment in the HIV-positive population is poorly documented. Small studies indicate that it is likely that the toxicity of radiotherapy and chemotherapy is increased. More frequent and more severe adverse reactions may compromise the patient's ability to complete the proposed treatment. This tendency may be greater in patients whose CD4 count is $<200/\mu L$ at the start of treatment. Multinational prospective randomised trials are ongoing in the developing world to establish the efficacy and toxicity of combined chemoradiotherapy in the HIV-positive population.

Kaposi's sarcoma

Kaposi's sarcoma (KS) is a low-grade vascular soft tissue sarcoma associated with human herpes virus 8. It is the malignancy most commonly associated with HIV infection, occurring in epidemic form in association with AIDS. Prior to the HIV pandemic, KS existed in a sporadic form in elderly men of Mediterranean origin and an endemic form in sub-Saharan Africa. Unlike epidemic KS, these diseases are indolent with predominantly cutaneous manifestations. All types of KS are far more common in men than in women.

Clinical features

The clinical course is variable, ranging from minimal symptoms and signs to widely disseminated disease involving multiple organs resulting in significant morbidity and mortality. Almost any organ may be involved; some of the commoner presenting symptoms are listed in Box 2.

Management

There is no known cure for KS. The aim of treatment is to palliate symptoms and to postpone disease progression.

All patients with KS should be commenced on HAART, which can induce tumour response. HAART can be given in combination with other treatments for KS.

Individual symptomatic lesions can be treated with a variety of techniques including intralesional injection of cytotoxics such as vinblastine, radiotherapy, laser therapy or cryotherapy.

Systemic therapy is reserved for those with diffuse disease, particularly those who have visceral involvement. Patients who have failed other treatments may also benefit. Liposomal preparations of doxorubicin and daunorubicin produce a similar response rate to combination chemotherapy regimens with an improved side effect profile, making these agents first line treatment for patients with access to these drugs.

Box 1 HIV infection and malignancy

AIDS-defining cancers
- Kaposi's sarcoma
- Non-Hodgkin's lymphoma
- Cervical cancer

Cancers associated with HIV infection
- Hodgkin's disease
- Anogenital malignancy
- Head and neck cancer
- Lung cancer
- Skin cancer
- Testicular cancer
- Squamous cell carcinoma of the conjunctiva (Fig. 1)

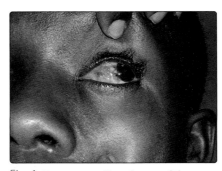

Fig. 1 **Squamous cell carcinoma of the conjunctiva** – an HIV-associated malignancy.

Box 2 Kaposi's sarcoma – presenting symptoms

- *Skin* – papular lesions of variable colour most commonly on lower limbs. Often associated with disproportionate lymphoedema
- *Oral cavity* – lesions usually on the palate where they may interfere with eating and become ulcerated due to trauma. Large lesions may obstruct the airway
- *Gastrointestinal tract* – nodules within the bowel may produce symptoms such as nausea and vomiting, pain, weight loss and obstruction
- *Respiratory system* – lesions within the lung may present with cough, haemoptysis and chest pain

Additional active cytotoxic drugs include vinca alkaloids, other anthracyclines, bleomycin and taxanes.

Lymphoma

Burkitt's lymphoma, immunoblastic lymphoma and primary lymphoma of the central nervous system are classified as AIDS-defining illnesses. Hodgkin's lymphoma is the most common of the HIV-associated cancers listed in Box 1. Treatment of these conditions in the HIV-positive patient is the same as that in the HIV-negative patient and is detailed in the relevant chapters.

Cervical cancer

HIV-positive women are more likely to have high-grade cervical intraepithelial neoplasia. Invasive cervical cancer presents at a younger age and is more resistant to treatment in this group. Increased recurrence rates, rapid progression to distant metastases and decreased survival in comparison with the HIV-negative population have been documented.

In the developed world, where women have access to HAART, cervical cancer is the most likely cause of death in an HIV-positive woman diagnosed with cervical cancer and it should be treated radically according to standard treatment regimens for HIV-negative women. Standard treatment is discussed in the chapter on cervical cancer.

In the developing world, cervical cancer is a huge public health issue. Screening programmes have been shown to be effective in the general population. The efficacy of such programmes, specifically in the treatment of premalignant lesions in HIV-positive women, remains to be elucidated. Many women have poor access to health facilities and receive little or no treatment for their disease.

Solid organ transplantation

The immunosuppressive therapy administered to prevent organ rejection after kidney or heart transplant is associated with an increased risk of certain cancers, as listed in Box 3. The risk of cancer is associated not only with the degree of immunosuppression but with coexisting causative factors such as viral agents (Epstein–Barr virus, human papilloma virus and human herpes virus 8) and sun exposure in the case of skin cancers. Cardiac transplant recipients are more immunosuppressed than renal transplant recipients as organ rejection is potentially fatal.

Skin cancer is the most common cancer in this group of patients. Squamous cell carcinoma is commoner than basal cell carcinoma, in contrast to the general population in whom basal cell carcinoma is more common. Other clinical differences are apparent in the transplant population; skin cancers are more likely to be multiple, to occur at a younger age and to behave in a more aggressive manner with increased recurrence rates after treatment. Other solid tumours presenting in this population may also behave in a more aggressive manner.

Standard surgery, chemotherapy and radiotherapy treatment is indicated for malignancy in post-transplant patients. Cessation or reduction of immunosuppressive therapy should be considered in renal transplant recipients.

Box 3 Solid organ transplantation and malignancy

- Skin cancer – predominantly squamous cell carcinoma
- Lymphoma
- Kaposi's sarcoma
- Anogenital cancer
- Renal cell cancer
- Solid tumours common in the general population also slightly increased

---

Immunosuppression and malignancy

- Kaposi's sarcoma is the most common cancer associated with HIV infection.
- Kaposi's sarcoma, cervical cancer and non-Hodgkin's lymphoma are classified as AIDS-defining illnesses.
- HIV-positive patients with a good performance status should receive the same cancer treatment as HIV-negative patients.
- Immunosuppressive therapy after renal and cardiac transplant is associated with an increased incidence of malignancy.
- Skin cancer is the most common cancer seen in renal and cardiac transplant recipients.
- Cancers in immunosuppressed patients tend to be more aggressive.

Clinical trials

Evidence-based medicine is central to modern oncology practice. The evidence base is continuously refined by the publication of ongoing clinical trials, requiring that the clinician remain actively engaged in continuing medical education to keep abreast of developments. Interpretation of the literature is a skill which requires both clinical knowledge of the disease in question and critical analysis of trial methodology. This chapter provides a summary of some of the issues relevant to interpretation of clinical trials.

Types of clinical trials

Different trials are designed to answer different types of clinical questions. Fig. 1 illustrates some of the commonly used trial designs. In addition, trials of new drugs are generally classified as follows:

- *Phase I trial.* This is the first time the drug is tested in humans. Usually, healthy volunteers take part in these trials. In the oncology setting, this is often inappropriate and patients with advanced disease refractory to conventional treatment are offered participation. Escalating doses of the drug are administered and side effects monitored, to establish the maximum tolerated dose (MTD) and record the dose limiting toxicities.
- *Phase II trial.* The optimal dose as defined in the phase I trial is administered to patients with the disease to establish efficacy by demonstrating disease response. The aims of phase I and phase II studies may be achieved simultaneously. These studies are usually single arm studies including a small number (i.e. <50) of patients.
- *Phase III trial.* Once the safety and efficacy of the drug are established, a phase III trial can be conducted. The safety and efficacy of the drug is now compared to a standard treatment. An example of a phase III trial is the randomised controlled trial.

Randomised controlled clinical trials (RCT)

A well-designed RCT is the gold standard when comparing a new treatment to the current standard treatment (referred to as the control). Designing a trial is a complex process incorporating clinical, statistical, ethical and economic considerations. All aspects of the trial are planned and documented in advance in the trial protocol. A poorly designed trial will not answer the clinical question posed and is a disservice to the patients who participate.

Some of the key issues in planning a clinical trial are as follows:

- *Sample size.* Deciding how many patients to recruit for the trial is both a scientific and a pragmatic decision. The sample size must be sufficient to ensure the power of the trial is adequate. Most new treatments show a moderate difference in effect compared to the standard treatment and a large number of patients may be required to reliably detect the difference. Cooperation between multiple centres is often necessary to recruit the required number of patients.
- *Randomisation.* The purpose of randomisation is to eliminate bias in the assignment of patients to different arms in the trial. Randomisation is ideally performed by staff not directly involved in the trial.
- *Blinding.* In a double-blind trial, neither the patient nor the physician is aware of which treatment the patient receives. This is rarely practical in oncology trials. In a single-blind trial the physician assessing the patient is unaware which treatment the patient has received.
- *Statistical considerations.* Statistical considerations are vital in a well-designed RCT. A statistician should be consulted early in the planning process.
- *Endpoints.* Primary endpoints are used to measure treatment efficacy, common examples being overall survival, disease-free survival or tumour response. Secondary endpoints may be toxicity or quality of life. How endpoints are to be defined and measured should be clearly laid down in the trial protocol.
- *Quality of the control arm.* Any new treatment should be compared to the best available treatment.
- *Ethical issues.* All clinical trials are subject to review by a local ethics committee, which ensures that the trial protocol conforms to international standards. Guidelines regarding medical research involving human subjects have been devised by the World Medical Association (the Declaration of Helsinki) and by the International Conference on Harmonization for Good Clinical Practice (ICHGCP).

Systematic review and meta-analysis

Systematic review and meta-analysis are indispensable tools to the practising physician trying to interpret the medical literature and apply the evidence to clinical practice. The review process collects and summarises a large amount of widely disseminated and often contradictory information and provides a succinct conclusion.

A systematic review combines information from all available trials relating to a particular clinical question, both published and unpublished. A meta-analysis is a systematic review which combines the numerical results from trials, reanalyses them and estimates an overall result, usually displayed in a box and whisker (or forest) plot (Fig. 2). This gives the advantage of analysing very large numbers of patients, often in the thousands. It would be very difficult to conduct a single randomised trial of that magnitude. A meta-analysis therefore has greater power to detect a moderate difference than a single RCT.

Conducting a review

The quality of a review or meta-analysis depends on the trials included in it. Several points must be taken into account when considering trials for inclusion:

- Trials of sufficiently good quality should be included. The criteria used to gauge the quality of trials should be clearly stated in the report.
- Differences in design quality and patient populations in the chosen

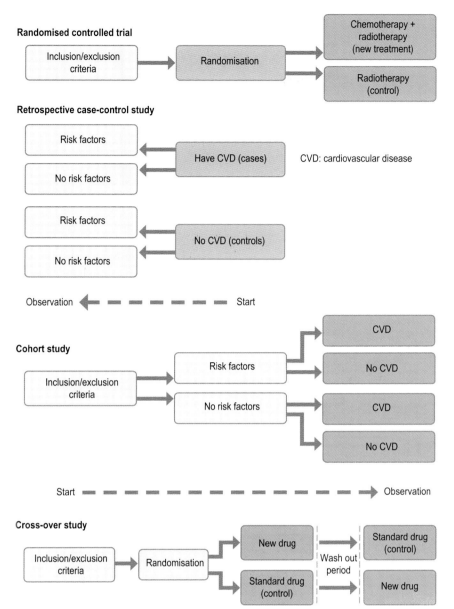

Fig. 1 **Common trial designs.**

trials may be impossible to avoid. There are various statistical measures which may be employed to overcome these differences. If these methods are used, it should be stated clearly in the report.

- Both published and unpublished data should be included to avoid publication bias. Publication bias refers to increased likelihood that positive results will be published, producing a bias in the literature.
- Ideally, original patient data should be procured with the cooperation of the original trial investigators. If this is not possible, summary statistics may be used.

The Cochrane Collaboration (www. cochrane.org) maintains a database of constantly updated reviews relating to all medical disciplines. International specialist organisations regularly produce reviews related to their particular interests; e.g. the Early Breast Cancer Trialists Group produce reviews relating to breast cancer treatment every 5 years.

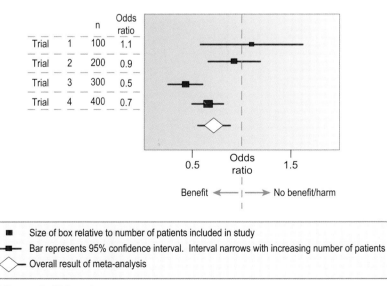

Fig. 2 **Box and whisker plot.**

> **Clinical trials**
>
> - The randomised controlled trial is the gold standard in trial design and forms the cornerstone of evidence-based medicine.
> - Most new oncology treatments provide a moderate benefit.
> - Trials must be powered to detect a moderate difference.
> - Systematic review and meta-analysis are valuable tools which provide a summary of large amounts of information, facilitating interpretation of the literature and application of the evidence to clinical practice.

Cancer screening

Effective screening for cancer is an invaluable public health measure. Healthy individuals are tested for an asymptomatic early stage of the disease which can then be treated, preventing progression to late stage disease and decreasing disease mortality.

Successful screening requires that the screening test, the disease in question and the screening programme fulfil certain criteria (Box 1). The applicability of screening to the commonest cancers is discussed below, with relevant points summarised in Table 1.

Screening programmes are applied to a target population, i.e. those at higher risk of developing the disease. A 'call and recall' system is employed to invite people for screening at calculated intervals. The screening test may detect premalignant disease or asymptomatic invasive disease.

Evidence-based cancer screening

Screening programmes in breast, cervical and colorectal cancer have been proven to reduce disease-specific mortality. Several types of bias may complicate screening research and

studies should be designed to take account of these issues:

- *Lead time bias.* Early diagnosis falsely appears to improve survival. The natural history of the disease is unchanged, but the time interval from diagnosis to death is longer because the disease is diagnosed earlier during an asymptomatic phase.
- *Length bias.* A screening programme is more likely to diagnose less aggressive disease. Aggressive cancers develop over a short period of time and are more likely to present with symptoms between rounds of screening. Less aggressive cancers progress more slowly and are picked up by the screening programme before they become symptomatic.
- *Selection bias.* People who attend for screening are likely to have better health outcomes. Those who attend appointments are more likely to look after their health than are those who do not attend. This may result in a biased population.
- *Verification bias.* The sensitivity and specificity of a screening programme can be biased because disease status is not verified in the entire population, only in those who test positive.

Sensitivity and specificity

Sensitivity is defined as the proportion of people with the disease who test positive on the screening test. Specificity is defined as the proportion of people who do not have the disease who test negative on the screening test. Ideally both of these figures should be as close to 100% as possible. However, the more sensitive a test is, the less likely it is to be highly specific and vice versa. In practice, a good screening test offers a compromise between the two. The potential results of a screening test are discussed in Box 2.

Breast cancer

Screening for breast cancer has been a controversial topic over the years, complicated by the interaction between medical and political interests. It is now accepted that mammogram-based screening saves lives.

The mammogram uses low energy X-rays to produce a picture of the breast with maximum contrast between normal tissue and changes characteristic of early malignancy or premalignant lesions.

Women with screen-detected abnormalities are referred to a specialist breast clinic for assessment and appropriate treatment. Screening has led to a large increase in the proportion of women diagnosed with ductal carcinoma in situ, providing new research challenges in determining optimal treatment. Invasive cancers diagnosed on screening are treated in the same way as cancers which present with symptoms.

In the UK, the breast cancer screening programme invites all women aged between 50 and 70 years

---

Box 1 Criteria for effective screening

The screening test
- High sensitivity and specificity
- Acceptable to the population
- Safe and validated in the population
- Economic

The disease
- Early stage is asymptomatic
- The natural history is well understood
- Treatment at the early stage alters the outcome
- Treatment at the late stage is associated with poorer outcome
- An important health problem

The screening programme
- Agreed policy based on high quality evidence-based diagnosis and treatment
- Should be proven to reduce mortality in a randomised controlled trial
- Adequate resources should be made available
- Health gain should outweigh morbidity of screening
- Cost-effective
- Should be monitored

Box 2 Results of a screening test

- *True positive* – the test is positive and the person has the disease.
- *True negative* – the test is negative and the person does not have the disease.
- *False positive* – the test is positive but the person does not have the disease. Detrimental psychological and economic effects are produced by unnecessary investigations.
- *False negative* – the test is negative but the person does have the disease. The diagnosis has been missed. The person may be diagnosed on the next round of screening or may present in the interval with symptomatic cancer.

Table 1 Summary of cancer screening recommendations for common cancers

Cancer	Target population	Screening test	Screening interval
Breast	Women aged 50–70 years	Mammography	3 years
Colorectal	Men and women aged 60–69 years	Faecal occult blood test	2 years
Lung	Not recommended		
Prostate	Not recommended		
Cervix	Women aged 25–64 years	Pap smear (cervical cytology)	3-yearly to age 49, 5-yearly to age 64

to come for screening every 3 years. Approximately 1.5 million women are screened annually at an estimated cost of £70–80 million.

Colorectal cancer

Regular screening with the faecal occult blood (FOB) test has been proven to reduce mortality from colorectal cancer. A positive FOB test prompts an invitation for colonoscopy, at which time a cancer or a polyp may be diagnosed.

In the UK, a national bowel cancer screening programme is currently undergoing a pilot phase. People aged 60–69 years of age will be screened every 2 years. A FOB test is sent to each person in the post. The test can be performed at home and returned to the test centre by post for reporting.

Cervical cancer

Screening for cervical intraepithelial neoplasia (CIN), a premalignant lesion of the cervix, effectively reduces the incidence of cervical cancer and the number of deaths due to cervical cancer. The national screening programme in the UK has now successfully achieved both of these goals, using a systematic call and recall system, which covers over 80% of the population, costing in the region of £130 million annually. Screening begins at 25 years and is offered 3-yearly to the age of 49 and 5-yearly to age 64.

The initial cervical cancer screening programmes instituted many years ago in the UK were unsuccessful, failing to show a reduction in disease-specific mortality. This was thought to be due to a failure to reach the population most at risk and to poor quality reporting, treatment and recall mechanisms, deficits which have been corrected in the current programme.

The screening test used is the Papanicolau smear (Pap smear), in which the cervix is scraped circumferentially to remove some cells which are then analysed by liquid-based cytology. CIN is illustrated in Fig. 1. Reporting mechanisms are subject to rigorous quality control systems.

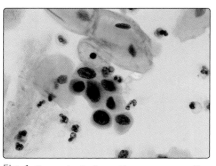

Fig. 1 **Severely dyskaryotic squamous cells consistent with high-grade CIN.** *Courtesy of Dr David Delaney.*

Screening for cervical cancer in the developing world

There is now a large disparity in the incidence of cervical cancer in developed and developing countries largely due to the success of screening and treatment programmes in the developed world. Implementation of screening programmes in low resource settings presents multifaceted difficulties ranging from lack of resources and expertise to practical difficulties such as the absence of postal addresses for most citizens.

The Pap smear, which requires laboratory facilities and a report from an experienced cytologist, presents difficulties for implementation of screening programmes in low resource settings. Visual inspection techniques have been used with some success in sub-Saharan Africa and India. These methods provide instant results, can be performed by trained nurses or midwives and do not require laboratory facilities.

- Visual inspection with acetic acid – 5% acetic acid solution is applied to the cervix. Premalignant lesions turn a white colour, easily seen with the naked eye.

- Visual inspection with Lugol's iodine – 5% Lugol's iodine solution is applied to the cervix. Normal tissue turns mahogany brown, premalignant lesions fail to take up the iodine.

Prostate cancer

Prostate specific antigen (PSA) is a tumour marker used in the diagnosis of prostate cancer. It is elevated in early stage disease; hence its potential attractiveness as a screening test. It has been used as a screening test alone or in combination with digital rectal examination. Men with a PSA level above a predetermined cut-off point are referred for investigation and undergo a prostate biopsy.

The efficacy of these approaches in reducing prostate cancer mortality has not yet been proven. Early stage prostate cancer is associated with prolonged survival and it is not yet clear whether mass screening using PSA will significantly reduce mortality. There is a large multinational, European trial ongoing aimed at answering this question.

National screening for prostate cancer is not recommended at present in the UK as several of the criteria listed in Box 1 have not been fulfilled. Men who are concerned about prostate cancer or who request a PSA test should be provided with sufficient information so that they can make an informed decision about having the test.

Lung cancer

The poor outcomes of treatment in advanced lung cancer make it a particularly attractive candidate for a successful screening programme. Unfortunately, various approaches using sputum cytology, chest radiographs or low-dose CT scans of the chest have not demonstrated a reduction in disease-specific mortality. At present, routine lung cancer screening is not recommended.

> ### Cancer screening
> - A successful screening test should be safe, acceptable and economic with a high sensitivity and specificity.
> - Screening for breast, cervical and colorectal cancer has been proven to reduce mortality from these diseases.
> - Screening for prostate and lung cancer has not yet been proven to reduce mortality from these diseases.
> - National screening programmes for breast and cervical cancer are operating in the UK using mammograms and cervical cytology, respectively.

Additional reading and sources of information

Reference textbooks

DeVita V T, Hellman S, Rosenberg S 2004 Cancer: Principles and Practice of Oncology, 7th edn. Lippincott Williams & Wilkins

Peckham M, Pinedo H, Veronesi U (eds) 1995 Oxford Textbook of Oncology. Oxford University Press

Tannock I F, Hill R P, Bristow R G, Harrington L 2004 The Basic Science of Oncology, 4th edn. McGraw-Hill

Useful links

International cancer research organisation

http://www.uicc.org/

National cancer research organisations

http://www.eacr.org/
http://www.iob.org/
http://www.icr.ac.uk/
http://www.ncri.org.uk/
http://www.lrf.org.uk/
http://www.mrc.ac.uk/index.htm
http://www.ntrac.org.uk/
http://info.cancerresearchuk.org/

Professional organisations

http://www.esmo.org/
http://www.baso.org/
http://www.rcog.org.uk/
http://www.rcr.ac.uk/

Patient care and advocacy organisations

http://www.cancerbackup.org.uk/Home
http://www.macmillan.org.uk/Home.aspx
http://www.mariecurie.org.uk/
https://www.teenagecancertrust.org/
http://www.mesothelioma.uk.com/

Glossary

Abdominoperineal resection – A surgical procedure in which the anus, rectum and part of the colon are removed along with a cancer. The anus is closed and the colon is brought out onto the skin as a colostomy.

Accelerated radiotherapy – The radiation dose is given over a shorter period of time than conventional treatment.

Acute toxicity – Side effects which occur immediately or shortly after treatment. In general these side effects reduce over time.

Adenocarcinoma – Cancer that arises in cells forming glandular type tissue. This type of tissue is present in many organs of the body.

Adenoma – A benign tumour.

Adjuvant treatment – Treatment given in addition to the primary treatment to decrease the likelihood of cancer recurrence and to increase the long-term survival. It is usually given after the primary treatment; for example, chemotherapy or radiotherapy given after surgery.

Adverse effect – An unwanted side effect of treatment.

Anastomosis – A connection of the cut ends of a hollow organ, e.g. connection of the bowel after a tumour has been removed.

Anterior resection – A surgical procedure in which part of the colon is removed along with a cancer. The cut ends of bowel are rejoined. The anus is left in place and the patient may pass stool normally after surgery.

Apoptosis – Also called programmed cell death. A series of steps occurring within the cell lead to its death. It is a normal mechanism within the body.

Chronic toxicity – Side effects which occur a long time after treatment. In general, these side effects are permanent, e.g. lung fibrosis due to chemotherapy or radiotherapy.

Combined modality therapy – A combination of two types of treatment, e.g. chemotherapy and radiotherapy.

Complete response (remission) – Complete disappearance of the tumour on clinical and radiological examination after treatment.

Concomitant chemotherapy – Chemotherapy which is given at the same time as radiotherapy. Also referred to as concurrent therapy.

CT scan – A detailed picture of the internal structures of the body taken using an X-ray machine linked to a computer which can reconstruct the picture.

Cytology – Looking at individual cells under a microscope.

Disease-free survival rate – The proportion of patients who remain alive without evidence of the disease in question.

Disease-free survival – Patients who are alive with no evidence of disease after a specified period of time. Also called relapse-free survival. Used to measure the outcome of treatment in clinical trials.

Disease-specific survival rate – The proportion of patients who remain alive with no evidence of the disease being studied. This does not take into account patients who have died of causes other than the disease in question.

Drug resistance/multidrug resistance – Changes in cancer cells make chemotherapy drugs less effective in killing the cancer cells.

False negative – *see* Sensitivity.

False positive – *see* Specificity.

Fractionation – Dividing the total dose of radiation into smaller doses conventionally given once a day, 5 days a week.

Hyperfractionation – Increasing the number of fractions compared to conventional treatment. This decreases the dose per fraction.

Hypofractionation – Decreasing the number of fractions compared to conventional treatment. This increases the dose per fraction.

Median survival time – The time at which half of the patients studied will still be alive.

Metastasis – A secondary tumour which has spread from a primary tumour in another part of the body.

MRI scan – Radiowaves and a powerful magnet are used to produce a detailed picture of the internal structures of the body. MRI is superior to CT scan in imaging the brain, nerves, spinal cord and soft tissues.

Multicentre trial – A trial that involves a number of different hospitals.

Multidisciplinary treatment – Treatment which involves specialists from a number of disciplines, typically surgical oncology, medical oncology and radiation oncology. Specialist nurses and disciplines such as physiotherapy and occupational therapy may also be involved.

Neoadjuvant – Treatment given in addition to the primary treatment but administered prior to primary treatment, e.g. chemotherapy or radiotherapy given prior to surgery. This may be done to reduce the size of the tumour and make it more amenable to curative surgery.

Occult disease – Malignant disease that is not evident by clinical examination or revealed by investigations.

Overall survival rate – The proportion of patients who remain alive. Death due to any cause is considered.

Palliative treatment – Treatment of any type that is intended to relieve the signs and symptoms of cancer and improve the patient's quality of life.

Partial response (remission) – A partial reduction in tumour size after treatment.

PET scan – Radioactive glucose is injected into a vein and taken up by active cells within the body. Many cancer cells take up a large amount of glucose. The radioactive emissions from the glucose can be used to produce a picture showing the location of the cancer cells.

Prognostic factors – Factors which have been proven to predict the long-term survival of patients, e.g. larger tumour size is associated with reduced cure in some cancer sites.

Progression – An increase in the size of the cancer or the appearance of new cancers in the body. May also refer to the progression of cancer symptoms.

Radical treatment – Treatment of any type that is intended to cure the cancer.

Radiosensitiser – A drug that increases the sensitivity of cells to radiotherapy. This increases the effect the radiotherapy has on cancer cells but may also increase the side effects.

Recurrence – Cancer which reappears after a period of complete response.

Refractory – In oncology, a cancer that is resistant to treatment.

Sensitivity – The proportion of patients with a disease who test positive for the disease. Patients with a disease who test negative for the disease are said to have a false negative test.

Specificity – The proportion of patients without a disease who test negative for a disease. No medical test is 100% specific – some patients will test positive. This is a false positive test.

Standard treatment/conventional treatment – Treatment that is widely accepted as the best currently available for a particular type of cancer based on the evidence of clinical trials.

Supportive therapy – Treatment aimed at relieving the patient's signs and symptoms.

Time to progression – The length of time from treatment to documentation of disease progression. Often used to monitor the effectiveness of treatment in clinical trials involving patients who have advanced cancer.

Toxicity – The side effects produced by treatment.

Subject index

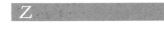